Curbside Consultation
in IBS

49 Clinical Questions

CURBSIDE CONSULTATION IN GASTROENTEROLOGY
SERIES

SERIES EDITOR, FRANCIS A. FARRAYE, MD, MSC

Curbside Consultation
in IBS

49 Clinical Questions

Brian E. Lacy, MD, PhD

Associate Professor of Medicine
Dartmouth Medical School
Director of the GI Motility Laboratory
Dartmouth-Hitchcock Medical Center
Lebanon, New Hampshire

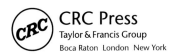

CRC Press
Taylor & Francis Group
Boca Raton London New York

CRC Press is an imprint of the
Taylor & Francis Group, an **informa** business

First published 2011 by SLACK Incorporated

Published 2024 by CRC Press
2385 NW Executive Center Drive, Suite 320, Boca Raton FL 33431

and by CRC Press
4 Park Square, Milton Park, Abingdon, Oxon, OX14 4RN

CRC Press is an imprint of Taylor & Francis Group, LLC

© 2011 Taylor & Francis Group, LLC

Library of Congress Cataloging-in-Publication Data

Curbside consultation in IBS : 49 clinical questions / [edited by] Brian E. Lacy.
    p. ; cm. -- (Curbside consultation in gastroenterology series)
  Irritable bowel syndrome
  Includes bibliographical references and index.
   ISBN 978-1-55642-985-9 (pbk.)
   1. Irritable colon--Miscellanea. I. Lacy, Brian E. II. Title: Irritable bowel syndrome. III. Series: Curbside consultation in gastroenterology.
   [DNLM: 1. Irritable Bowel Syndrome. WI 520]
   RC862.I77C87 2011
   616.3'42--dc22
                              2011010164

ISBN: 9781556429859 (pbk)
ISBN: 9781003523574 (ebk)

DOI: 10.1201/9781003523574

Dedication

This book is dedicated to two groups of people. First, to my co-authors, who willingly, enthusiastically, and cheerfully somehow found the time in their incredibly busy lives to write a state-of-the art chapter on their specialty within the field of IBS. Your tireless efforts to expand the boundaries of knowledge in the field of IBS and to improve patient care are greatly appreciated by everyone in the discipline of medicine.

Second, on behalf of all of my co-authors, this book is dedicated to all of our patients who suffer from IBS. We hope that the information presented in this book will provide you and your physicians with information that will improve your symptoms and your quality of life.

To make this book interactive, and to keep readers of the book as up-to-date as possible on new developments in the field of IBS, a website will be available:

http://www.curbsideconsultations.com/gastro/IBS

Each month, an additional new IBS consult question will be posted and readers can pose questions (and answers) to the editor and authors.

Contents

Acknowledgments

Writing and editing a book requires the combined efforts of many people who work tirelessly behind the scenes, often without credit. To counteract that, I would like to thank my acquisitions editor at SLACK Incorporated, Carrie Kotlar. This book never would have come to fruition without her tireless efforts. In addition, I would like to thank the project editor, who did a wonderful job blending the many different writing styles of all of the authors to form a coherent theme. I would also like to thank Dr. Francis Farraye, the series editor for the *Curbside Consultation in GI Series*, who recognized the need for this book, and who spent innumerable hours helping to coordinate this project. Finally, I would like to thank my family, Elaine, Colin, and Hannah, for their unwavering support during this project.

About the Editor

Brian E. Lacy, PhD, MD is currently an Associate Professor of Medicine at Dartmouth Medical School, and Director of the GI Motility Laboratory at the Dartmouth-Hitchcock Medical Center in Lebanon, New Hampshire.

Dr. Lacy's clinical and basic science research interests focus on disorders of gastrointestinal motility, with an emphasis on irritable bowel syndrome, dyspepsia, gastroparesis, acid reflux disease, constipation, intestinal pseudo-obstruction, achalasia, and visceral pain. He is the author of numerous articles and textbook chapters on gastrointestinal motility disorders and functional bowel disorders. Dr. Lacy is a reviewer for a number of scientific journals and is a member of a number of different scientific organizations, including the American College of Gastroenterology, the American Gastroenterology Association, the American Motility Society, and the Functional Brain-Gut Research Group. Dr. Lacy is the co-author of a book for the general public on acid reflux disease, *Healing Heartburn,* and is the author of *Making Sense of IBS,* a book for the general public on irritable bowel syndrome.

Dr. Lacy received his doctorate in cell biology from Georgetown University in Washington, DC, and his medical degree from the University of Maryland in Baltimore. Dr. Lacy was a resident in internal medicine at the Dartmouth-Hitchcock Medical Center in Lebanon, NH, where he continued his training as Chief Resident and as a Fellow in Gastroenterology. He is board certified in both internal medicine and gastroenterology.

Contributing Authors

Giovanni Barbara, MD (Question 8)
Assistant Professor of Medicine
Department of Clinical Medicine
St. Orsola-Malpighi Hospital
University of Bologna
Bologna, Italy

Adil E. Bharucha, MD, MBBS (Question 28)
Professor of Medicine
Division of Gastroenterology and Hepatology
Mayo Clinic
Rochester, Minnesota

Steven J. Bollipo, MBBS, FRACP
Director of Gastroenterology & Endoscopy
John Hunter Hospital
Newcastle, NSW, Australia

Michael Camilleri, MD (Question 49)
Professor of Medicine and Physiology
Mayo Clinic College of Medicine
Director, Clinical Enteric Neuroscience
Translational Epidemiological Research
Rochester, Minnesota

Brooks D. Cash, MD, FACP, FACG, AGAF (Question 7)
Professor of Medicine
Uniformed Services University of the Health Sciences
Chief of Medicine
National Naval Medical Center
Bethesda, Maryland

Joseph Y. Chang, MD, MPH (Question 22)
Mayo Clinic
Rochester, Minnesota

Lin Chang, MD (Question 17)
Professor of Medicine in Residence
UCLA Department of Medicine, Division of Digestive Diseases
David Geffen School of Medicine, UCLA
Co-Director, UCLA Center for Neurovisceral Sciences and Women's Health (CNS/WH)
Los Angeles, California

Rok Seon Choung, MD, PhD (Question 1)
Assistant Professor of Medicine
Division of Gastroenterology and Hepatology
Mayo Clinic
Rochester, Minnesota

Filippo Cremonini, MD, MSc, PhD (Question 10)
Instructor in Medicine
Harvard Medical School
Director, Translational Research Motility Center
Beth Israel Deaconess Medical Center
Division of Gastroenterology
Boston, Massachusetts

Michael D. Crowell, PhD, FACG, AGAF (Question 3)
Professor of Medicine
CTSA Education Director MCA
Consultant
Division of Gastroenterology and Hepatology
Co-Director, GI Physiology and Motility
Mayo Clinic
Scottsdale, Arizona

Douglas A. Drossman, MD (Question 48)
Co-Director, UNC Center for Functional GI
& Motility Disorders
Professor of Medicine and Psychiatry
University of North Carolina at Chapel
Hill
Chapel Hill, North Carolina

Ronnie Fass, MD, FACP, FACG (Question 24)
Professor of Medicine
University of Arizona
Chief of Gastroenterology
Head Neuroenteric Clinical Research Group
Southern Arizona VA Health Care System
Section of Gastroenterology
Tucson, Arizona

*Fernando Fernández-Bañares, MD, PhD
(Question 31)*
Department of Gastroenterology
Hospital Universitari Mútua Terrassa
Terrassa, Spain

Alexander Ford, MD (Question 34)
Leeds Gastroenterology Institute
Leeds General Infirmary
Leeds, United Kingdom

*Amy E. Foxx Orenstein, DO, FACG, FACP
(Question 6)*
Associate Professor of Medicine
Division of Gastroenterology and Hepatology
Mayo Clinic
Scottsdale, Arizona

*Elizabeth A. Friedlander, PhD, ANP-C, FNP
(Question 44)*
Division of Gastroenterology
Beth Israel Deaconess Medical Center
Boston, Massachusetts

*Christine Frissora, MD, FACG, FACP
(Question 30)*
Associate Professor of Medicine
The Joan Sanford I. Weill Medical College
of Cornell University
Assistant Attending Physician
NewYork-Presbyterian Hospital Cornell
Campus
New York, New York

Larissa Fujii, MD (Question 3)
Department of Internal Medicine
Mayo Clinic
Scottsdale, Arizona

Madhusudan Grover, MD (Questions 6, 48)
Instructor in Medicine
Division of Gastroenterology and Hepatology
Mayo Clinic College of Medicine
Rochester, Minnesota

Kok-Ann Gwee, FRCP, PhD (Question 18)
Adjunct Associate Professor of Medicine
Yong Loo Lin School of Medicine
National University of Singapore
Gastroenterologist
Gleneagles Hospital
Singapore

Albena Halpert, MD (Question 29)
Assistant Professor
Section of Gastroenterology
Boston University School of Medicine
Boston, Massachusetts

Lucinda A. Harris, MD (Questions 3, 38)
Associate Professor of Medicine
Division of Gastroenterology and Hepatology
Mayo Clinic
Scottsdale, Arizona

Margaret M. Heitkemper, PhD, RN, FAAN (Question 17)
Professor and Chairperson
Department of Biobehavioral Nursing and Health Systems
Adjunct Professor
Division of Gastroenterology
University of Washington School of Medicine
Seattle, Washington

Tiberiu Hershcovici, MD (Chapter 24)
Research Fellow in Gastroenterology
University of Arizona Health Sciences Center
Tucson, Arizona

Lesley A. Houghton, PhD, FSB, FACG, AGAF (Question 13)
Professor of Medicine, College of Medicine
Director of Research, Gastroenterology and Hepatology
Mayo Clinic
Jacksonville, Florida
University of Manchester
Translational Medicine
Manchester, United Kingdom

Basma Issa, MD, MPhil (Question 45)
Research Associate
Neurogastroenterology Unit
Wythenshawe Hospital
The University of Manchester
Manchester, United Kingdom

John E. Kellow, MD, FRACP (Question 12)
Associate Professor and Head of the Discipline of Medicine
Northern Clinical School
University of Sydney
Gastroenterologist and Director of the Gastrointestinal Investigation Unit
Royal North Shore Hospital
Sydney, Australia

David Klibansky, MD (Question 16)
Dartmouth-Hitchcock Medical Center
Lebanon, New Hampshire

Jeff Lackner, PsyD (Question 46)
Associate Professor
Department of Medicine
Behavioral Medicine Clinic
State University of New York at Buffalo School of Medicine
Buffalo, New York

Anthony Lembo, MD (Question 44)
Associate Professor of Medicine
Harvard Medical School
Division of Gastroenterology
Beth Israel Deaconess Medical Center
Boston, Massachusetts

L. Campbell Levy, MD (Question 20)
Division of Gastroenterology and Hepatology
Dartmouth-Hitchcock Medical Center
Lebanon, New Hampshire

Rona L. Levy, MSW, PhD, MPH, AGAF, FACG (Question 2)
Professor and Director
Behavioral Medicine Research Group
University of Washington
Seattle, Washington

G. Richard Locke, MD (Question 1)
Professor of Medicine
Division of Gastroenterology and Hepatology
Mayo Clinic
Rochester, Minnesota

Burr Loew, MD (Question 43)
Dartmouth-Hitchcock Medical Center
Lebanon, New Hampshire

Susan Lucak, MD (Question 26)
Columbia University
New York, New York

Tisha N. Lunsford, MD (Question 38)
Assistant Professor of Medicine
Division of Gastroenterology and Hepatology
University of Texas Health Science Center
San Antonio, Texas

Juan Malagelada, MD (Question 14)
Chief, Gastroenterology Department
Professor of Digestive Diseases
Hospital Universitari Vall d'Hebron
Autonomous University of Barcelona
Barcelona, Spain

Kalyani Meduri, MD (Question 5)
Research Fellow
Neurogastroenterology & GI Motility
Research
University of Iowa Hospitals and Clinics
Iowa City, Iowa

Anil Minocha, MD, FACP, FACG (Question 32)
Professor of Medicine
Medical Service (IIIG)
VA Medical Center
Shreveport, Louisiana

Paul Moayyedi, BSc, MB, ChB, PhD, MPH, FRCP, FRCPC, AGAF, FACG (Question 35)
Co-Editor in Chief, *American Journal of Gastroenterology*
Director, Division of Gastroenterology
Professor of Medicine
McMaster University
Hamilton, Ontario, Canada

Rupa Mukherjee, MD (Question 26)
Fellow in Gastroenterology
Division of Digestive and Liver Diseases
Columbia University Medical Center
New York, New York

Agata Mulak, MD, PhD (Question 15)
UCLA Center for Neurobiology of Stress
David Geffen School of Medicine at UCLA
CURE: Digestive Diseases Research Center
VA Greater Los Angeles Healthcare System
Los Angeles, California

Richard Nahas, MD, CCFP (Question 47)
Medical Director, Seekers Centre for Integrative Medicine
Assistant Professor, Department of Family Medicine
Undergraduate Curriculum Content Expert
University of Ottawa
Ottawa, Canada

Kevin W. Olden, MD (Question 16)
Professor of Medicine and Psychiatry
Division of GI
University of Southern Alabama
Mobile, Alabama

Peter Paine, MD, PhD, MRCP (Question 13)
Department of Gastroenterology
Salford Royal NHS Foundation Trust
Salford, United Kingdom

Mark Pimentel, MD (Question 21)
Director, GI Motility Program
Cedars-Sinai Medical Center
Los Angeles, California

Eamonn M. M. Quigley, MD, FRCP, FACP, FACG, FRCPI (Question 42)
Professor of Medicine and Human Physiology
National University of Ireland, Cork
Cork, Ireland

Chris Radziwon, PhD (Question 46)
Post-Doctoral Fellow
Department of Medicine
Behavioral Medicine Clinic
State University of New York at Buffalo
School of Medicine
Buffalo, New York

Satish S. C. Rao, MD, PhD, FACG, AGAF, FRCP (Question 5)
Professor
Director, Neurogastroenterology/GI Motility
University of Iowa Carver College of Medicine
Division of GI
Iowa City, Iowa

Yehuda Ringel, MD (Question 41)
Associate Professor of Medicine
Division of Gastroenterology and Hepatology
University of North Carolina School of Medicine
Chapel Hill, North Carolina

Gisela Ringström, RN, PhD (Question 9)
Head Nurse
Section of Gastroenterology & Hepatology
Department of Internal Medicine
Sahlgrenska University Hospital
Gothenburg, Sweden

Yuri A. Saito-Loftus, MD, MPH (Question 22)
Assistant Professor of Medicine
Division of Gastroenterology and Hepatology
Mayo Clinic Rochester
Rochester, Minnesota

Lawrence R. Schiller, MD, FACP, FACG (Question 39)
Program Director
Gastroenterology Fellowship
Baylor University Medical Center
Dallas, Texas

Max J. Schmulson, MD (Question 25)
Profesor Titular de Medicina
Laboratorio de Hígado, Páncreas y Motilidad (HIPAM)
Departamento de Medicina Experimental
Facultad de Medicina
Universidad Nacional Autónoma de México-UNAM
Hospital General de México
México

Philip Schoenfeld, MD, MSEd, MSc (Epi) (Question 37)
Director, Training Program in GI Epidemiology
Associate Professor of Medicine
University of Michigan School of Medicine
Ann Arbor, Michigan

Ankur Sheth, MD, MPH, FACP, CNSC (Question 32)
Assistant Professor of Medicine
Louisiana State University Health Sciences Center
Shreveport, Louisiana

Lisa Shim, MB BS, FRACP (Question 12)
Research Fellow
Department of Gastroenterology
Royal North Shore Hospital
University of Sydney
St. Leonards, New South Wales
Australia

Corey A. Siegel, MD (Question 20)
Dartmouth-Hitchcock Medical Center
Gastroenterology and Hepatology
Lebanon, New Hampshire

Magnus Simrén, MD, PhD (Question 9)
Professor of Gastroenterology
Department of Internal Medicine
Institute of Medicine
Sahlgrenska Academy
University of Gothenburg
Gothenburg, Sweden

Ami D. Sperber, MD, MSPH (Question 19)
Department of Gastroenterology
Tel-Aviv Medical Center
Emeritus Professor of Medicine
Faculty of Health Sciences
Ben-Gurion University of the Negev
Beer-Sheva, Israel

Brennan Spiegel, MD (Question 11)
Assistant Professor of Medicine
VA Greater Los Angeles Healthcare System
David Geffen School of Medicine at UCLA
Director, UCLA/VA Center for Outcomes
Research and Education
Los Angeles, California

Vincenzo Stanghellini, MD (Question 8)
Professor of Medicine
Department of Clinical Medicine
St. Orsola-Malpighi Hospital
University of Bologna
Bologna, Italy

Yvette Taché, PhD (Question 15)
Professor of Medicine
David Geffen School of Medicine at UCLA
Director, CURE: Digestive Diseases
Research Center—Animal Core
Co-Director, Center for Neurovisceral
Sciences & Women's Health
VA Greater Los Angeles Healthcare System
Los Angeles, California

Jan Tack, MD, PhD (Question 36)
Professor of Medicine
Department of Gastroenterology
University Hospitals Leuven
Chair, Department of Pathophysiology
University of Leuven
Leuven, Belgium

Nicholas J. Talley, MD, PhD, FACP, FRACP, FRCP (Question 4)
Chair, Department of Internal Medicine
Mayo Clinic
Professor of Medicine and Epidemiology
Mayo Clinic College of Medicine
Consultant, Division of Gastroenterology
& Hepatology
Jacksonville, Florida

W. Grant Thompson, MD, FRCPC (Question 33)
Emeritus Professor of Medicine
Division of Gastroenterology
University of Ottawa
Ottawa, Canada

Kirsten T. Weiser, MD, MPH (Question 27)
Asheville Gastroenterology
Asheville, North Carolina

Peter J. Whorwell, BSc, MB, BS, MD, PhD, FRCP (Question 45)
Professor of Medicine and Gastroenterology
Neurogastroenterology Unit
Wythenshawe Hospital
The University of Manchester
Manchester, United Kingdom

Foreword

Optimum management of patients with IBS requires knowledge of such diverse and rapidly expanding information that busy practitioners often have trouble keeping up. This comprehensive, up-to-date book by many of the most experienced clinicians and knowledgeable researchers worldwide addresses this need. It clearly explains the epidemiology of IBS, its typical symptoms and associated disorders, accurate diagnosis, the heterogeneous pathophysiology, and effective therapies. The book is a valuable aid for generalists who care for children or adults, psychotherapists, gastroenterologists, and other specialists who help patients cope with this complex disorder.

George F. Longstreth, MD
Head of Gastroenterology, Kaiser Permanente
Clinical Professor of Medicine, UCSD School of Medicine
San Diego, California

Introduction

Irritable bowel syndrome (IBS) is one of the most common medical conditions found throughout the world. In the United States, it is estimated to affect 10% to 12% of adults. IBS symptoms are responsible for approximately 12% to 14% of all primary care office visits and are among the most common reasons for referral to a gastroenterologist. In fact, at least one-third of referrals to gastroenterologists are for the evaluation and management of IBS. The impact of IBS on both patients and society is well known. Irritable bowel syndrome significantly reduces the quality of life of those patients who suffer from the many symptoms of IBS, more so than common organic disorders, such as asthma and migraine headaches. In addition, IBS imposes a significant economic impact on our healthcare system. Current estimates are that we spend at least $10 billion per year in the United States evaluating, diagnosing, and treating symptoms of IBS. Surprisingly, despite its prevalence and impact to our healthcare system, significant misconceptions remain about IBS. For example, many patients mistakenly believe that IBS turns into cancer and that few or no treatments exist for their IBS symptoms, while many clinicians still focus their treatment only on the use of fiber.

During the past several years, significant changes have occurred in the field of IBS. New information is available regarding the value of dietary interventions for IBS symptoms. The use and utility of diagnostic testing has been carefully scrutinized. Advances have been made in our understanding of the etiology and pathophysiology of IBS, and new medications have been approved to ameliorate symptoms. These dramatic changes in this active field of clinical and basic science research highlight the need for an easy-to-use book for the busy clinician. *Curbside Consultation in IBS* is designed to provide you with up-to-date answers to the most commonly asked questions about the etiology, pathophysiology, diagnosis, and treatment of IBS.

The book is divided into 6 sections: the epidemiology and natural history of IBS, the diagnosis and impact of IBS, the pathophysiology of IBS, the association of IBS with other medical conditions, the treatment of IBS, and future therapies for IBS. The 49 chapters that make up this book have been written by the world's experts. Each section is designed to stand on its own, and the individual chapters in each section can be read as a group for a comprehensive review in that area. Alternatively, if pressed for time or if you need the answer to a very specific question, each chapter can be read individually, as if you were posing a question to an expert in the field of IBS. Finally, many readers will want to read the book from cover to cover, as *Curbside Consultation in IBS* serves as a timely reference for those who want a thorough review on this complex topic.

On behalf of all of the authors who contributed their extensive expertise to this edition of *Curbside Consultation in IBS*, we hope that this book answers your questions and allows you to better manage your patients with IBS.

> To make this book interactive, and to keep readers of the book as up-to-date as possible on new developments in the field of IBS, a website will be available: http://www.curbsideconsultations.com/gastro/IBS
>
> Each month, an additional new IBS consult question will be posted and readers can pose questions (and answers) to the editor and authors.

SECTION I

EPIDEMIOLOGY AND NATURAL HISTORY

How Common Is IBS?

G. Richard Locke III MD and Rok Seon Choung, MD

Irritable bowel syndrome (IBS) is a common functional gastrointestinal disorder that is characterized by symptoms of abdominal pain or discomfort and symptoms of diarrhea or constipation or both.[1-3] For chronic conditions, the best way to estimate how common they are is to report the number of people with the condition, which is the prevalence. In contrast, the incidence is the number of new cases, which is a better estimate for short-lived diagnoses. Generally, IBS is considered a highly prevalent functional gastrointestinal disorder. However, IBS epidemiology varies considerably according to the definition used. For example, the earlier Manning criteria are more generous and less restrictive than the recent Rome criteria. The range of IBS prevalence is from 3% to 25%, with most studies reporting results between 5% and 15% depending on the definition applied.

In a comprehensive review of the epidemiology of IBS in North America in 2002,[4] the prevalence estimates for IBS in the United States ranged from 3% to 20%. Because of the applied definition of IBS, the prevalence of IBS varied; that is, the more sensitive the definition, the higher the prevalence. In contrast, the more specific the definition, the lower the prevalence. This study also showed that the IBS prevalence decreased slightly with age, and the prevalence in women was slightly higher (2:1 female-to-male predominance). To place these figures in the proper context, it is important to note that this study was performed before the development of the Rome II criteria.

In more recent studies of the epidemiology of IBS in the US or Canada using Rome II criteria, the prevalence of IBS has been estimated to be 5% to 12%. In another systemic review of IBS in 2007, which was based on 13 studies in European Union nations, the prevalence of IBS was approximately 4% based on Rome II criteria. Similar to the North American data described above, there was a 2:1 female:male predominance. In Asia, the prevalence of IBS using the Rome II criteria has been reported to be 4% to 15%. Across Asia, the prevalence of IBS is higher in younger age groups. Interestingly, the female predominance reported in the West has not been reported in Asian countries. Notably, a higher prevalence of IBS in males has been reported in some Asian countries. Overall, the prevalence of IBS has been reported to be between 2% and 15% from Western countries or Asia, and IBS patients were more frequently younger in age. Female predominance is more prevalent in Western or tertiary hospital care settings.

In regard to IBS bowel habit subtypes, one systematic review reported[5] that population-based studies from the United States (Manning) found similar distributions among constipation-predominant IBS (IBS-C), diarrhea-predominant IBS (IBS-D), and IBS alternating between diarrhea and constipation (IBS-A). In contrast, European studies (Rome I, Rome II, or self-reporting) showed either IBS-C or IBS-A as the most prevalent subtypes. For example, in this study, approximately 16% of the IBS patients had IBS-C, 21% had IBS-D, and 63% had IBS-A.[5]

The incidence of IBS is not easy to determine because IBS may develop slowly and people may not seek care.[6] From a population-based study in the United States, which was based on two surveys sent to a random sample of people about 1 year apart, the IBS onset rate was 9%. However, in another study based on physician-based IBS diagnosis in the same population, the incidence rate of clinically diagnosed IBS was much lower, 196 cases per 100,000 person-years.[7] A study from Europe showed a similar incidence rate of IBS, about 200 to 300 per 100,000 people.[8] The fact that IBS symptoms may come and go and change over time further complicates the accurate determination of IBS incidence.[9] Thus, the 9% onset rate may have occurred in people who had IBS sometime in the past. Further complicating an accurate calculation of incidence is the fact that many people with IBS in the community do not seek care. The incidence of a clinical diagnosis of IBS is thus likely an underestimate. Nonetheless, if only half seek care, we can double the incidence to 400 per 100,000 per year and then multiply by 20-year disease duration to arrive at a prevalence of 12%, which is in keeping with the data.

The epidemiology of IBS can also be reviewed by evaluating specific causes of IBS. As described in other chapters (see Chapters 12 and 13), IBS is a multifactorial condition resulting from a number of different mechanisms such as disordered motility, visceral hypersensitivity, abnormal central processing, psychological factors, genetic factors, gut inflammation, and dietary factors. For example, between 5% and 30% of patients who suffer an acute episode of infectious gastroenteritis develop irritable bowel syndrome despite clearance of the inciting pathogen. From a systematic review of the post-infectious IBS, the incidence rate of IBS in patients with acute GI infection has been reported to be 10% (95% CI: 9.4 to 85.6).[10] In that study, post-infectious IBS was associated with younger age and anxious or depressed conditions.

Because IBS is primarily an ambulatory care issue, the epidemiology of IBS can also be evaluated by measuring clinic visits. IBS accounts for 10% to 15% of primary care visits and 25% to 50% of gastroenterology referral visits.[11] Data from the National Disease and Therapeutic Index (NDTI) showed that IBS accounts for 2.6 million office-based visits and 3.5 million all-location physician visits.[12] Recent data from the National Ambulatory Medical Care Survey (NAMCS) showed that IBS-related visits occurred at the same rate as for asthma and at 2.6 times the rate of visits for migraines.[13] Specialist consultations for IBS were of similar frequency to those for migraine but were more frequent than asthma.[13] More diagnostic and screening tests were ordered for IBS-related visits than for migraine- or asthma-related visits, and prescription rates were similar for all three conditions.

Finally, IBS can be disruptive to the personal and professional lives of those with IBS.[3] One population-based survey has shown that disability from IBS is high—patients miss an average of 13.4 days of work or school per year compared to 4.9 days per year for controls.[14] Measurement of health-related quality of life has also been shown to be lower in patients with IBS than in the US general population.[15]

Summary

IBS is a common condition affecting about 10% of the population. The incidence rate of IBS is 200 per 100,000 people but could be as high as 30% of the population in specific situations, such as after an acute gastrointestinal infection. Chapter 11 discusses the impact of this highly prevalent medical disorder.

References

1. Longstreth GF. Definition and classification of irritable bowel syndrome: current consensus and controversies. *Gastroenterol Clin North Am.* 2005;34:173-187.
2. Thompson W. Irritable bowel syndrome: pathogenesis and management. *Lancet.* 1993;341(8860): 1569-1572.
3. Longstreth GF, Thompson WG, Chey WD, Houghton LA, Mearin F, Spiller RC. Functional bowel disorders. *Gastroenterology.* 2006;130:1480-1491.
4. Saito YA, Schoenfeld P, Locke GR III. The epidemiology of irritable bowel syndrome in North America: a systematic review. *Am J Gastroenterol.* 2002;97:1910-1915.
5. Guilera M, Balboa A, Mearin F. Bowel habit subtypes and temporal patterns in irritable bowel syndrome: systematic review. *Am J Gastroenterol.* 2005;100:1174-1184.
6. Cremonini F, Talley NJ. Irritable bowel syndrome: epidemiology, natural history, health care seeking and emerging risk factors. *Gastroenterol Clin North Am.* 2005;34:189-204.
7. Locke GR III, Yawn BP, Wollan PC, Melton LJ III, Lydick E, Talley NJ. Incidence of a clinical diagnosis of the irritable bowel syndrome in a United States population. *Aliment Pharmacol Ther.* 2004;19(9):1025-1031.
8. Ruigomez A, Wallander M, Johansson S, Garcia Rodriguez L. One-year follow-up of newly diagnosed irritable bowel syndrome patients. *Aliment Pharmacol Ther.* 1999;13(8):1097-1102.
9. Halder SL, Locke GRI, Schleck CD, Zinsmeister A, Melton LJI, Talley NJ. Natural history of functional gastrointestinal disorders: A 12-year longitudinal population-based study. *Gastroenterology.* 2007;133(3):799-807.
10. Thabane M, Kottachchi D, Marshall J. Systematic review and meta-analysis: the incidence and prognosis of post-infectious irritable bowel syndrome. *Aliment Pharmacol Ther.* 2007;26:535-544.
11. Talley N, Zinsmeister AR, Van Dyke C, Melton LJ III. Epidemiology of colonic symptoms and the irritable bowel syndrome. *Gastroenterology.* 1991;101:927-934.
12. Sandler RS. Epidemiology of irritable bowel syndrome in the United States. *Gastroenterology.* 1990;99: 409-415.
13. Kozma C, Barghout V, Slaton T, Frech F, Reeder C. A comparison of office-based physician visits for irritable bowel syndrome and for migraine and asthma. *Managed Care Interface.* 2002;15:40-43.
14. Drossman DA, Li Z, Andruzzi E, et al. U.S. householder survey of functional gastrointestinal disorders. Prevalence, sociodemography, and health impact. *Dig Dis Sci.* 1993;38(9):1569-1580.
15. Gralnek IM, Hays RD, Kilbourne A, Naliboff B, Mayer EA. The impact of irritable bowel syndrome on health-related quality of life. *Gastroenterology.* 2000;119(3):654-660.

WHAT FACTORS ARE ASSOCIATED WITH IBS AND FUNCTIONAL ABDOMINAL PAIN IN CHILDREN?

Rona L. Levy, MSW, PhD, MPH, AGAF, FACG

Is there something in children's families that causes them to have irritable bowel syndrome (IBS) or other functional abdominal pain symptoms? If so, what are the recommendations for families to prevent or eliminate functional abdominal pain?

Based on the work of our group at the University of Washington and others who have been looking at how familial factors may be related to children's functional abdominal pain, the brief answer to the question of whether families cause functional abdominal pain is "sometimes." This chapter will give an overview of what is known about these questions and suggest strategies to address pediatric functional abdominal pain.

The possibility of family influence on functional abdominal pain was supported several years ago by a study from our group, which evaluated the amount of medical care and reasons for care received by children of IBS patients compared to children of parents who had not been treated for IBS. We found children of IBS patients sought health care significantly more than children of non-IBS patients. This finding was true not only for lower gastrointestinal problems, but for overall health-care services as well. Outpatient health-care costs over the 3-year period studied were also significantly higher for children of IBS parents than other children.

These findings suggested to us one of two possibilities: either children inherited something from their parents that brought about these similar illness patterns or children were somehow learning to have illness experiences similar to their parents. Therefore, we conducted a study of identical twins to determine the rate of IBS among identical and nonidentical twins and their parents. The findings of this study were quite interesting. We studied more than 6000 families and found that the probability of having IBS is significantly greater if you have an identical twin with IBS rather than a nonidentical twin. In other words, this study found *some* evidence for a genetic contribution to IBS.

However, there was an even more intriguing finding in this study: The rates of IBS between (a) mothers and twins were significantly higher than the rates between (b) two nonidentical twins. Because these two sets should share the same number of genes, you would expect these numbers to be equal if parent-child learning were not a factor. Based on these significant differences, we concluded that there was very likely a social learning contribution to the development of IBS as well. Thus, as we concluded in our abstract, "Heredity contributes to development of irritable bowel syndrome, but social learning (what an individual learns from those in his or her environment) has an equal *or greater* influence."[1]

Pursuing a related line of work at Vanderbilt University, Dr. Lynn Walker's group found patterns of gastrointestinal symptoms and psychological traits in the **families** of child functional abdominal pain patients that were similar to those in the child patients themselves. This led her to suspect that patients could be learning some of their responses from their family members. Parents' psychological distress also seemed to be predictive of a child's ability to recover from functional abdominal pain.

Walker's group also has investigated how a number of child psychological traits may be related to functional abdominal pain. For example, children whose parents were overly protective or critical of their pain often experienced more impairment or somatic symptoms. This was particularly true of those children who were already at risk for difficulties due to higher levels of emotional distress. Also, life stress predicted symptom maintenance in functional abdominal pain patients even up to 5 years following their medical evaluation.[2]

Our group next turned its attention to trying to figure out what exactly might be going on between parents and children to account for some of these observations. We started with a basic principle of learning theory: behavior that is rewarded is more likely to occur in the future. We looked at the responses of parents to children's symptom complaints to see if the level of rewarding responses was related to the level of symptom complaints. To add another level of interest, we also decided to look separately at mothers with IBS and mothers without IBS to see if these two groups of mothers responded differently to their children. We found parent solicitousness in response to children's symptom complaints (as well as parent IBS status) was related to children's symptom reporting, clinic visits, and illness-related school absenteeism. Figure 2-1 illustrates this finding for school absences.[3]

A next logical step in this line of inquiry was to determine if children's disability and symptom reports could be reduced by an intervention. Our study used a cognitive behavioral intervention (ie, Social Learning and Cognitive Behavioral Therapy [SLCBT]) aimed at providing parents and children with a set of skills that included different ways for them both to respond to children's symptoms. In a recently published study, we reported the results of this study of 200 children and their parents. We found children in the cognitive behavioral condition showed greater baseline to follow-up decreases in pain and GI symptom severity than children in the comparison condition. Also, parents in the cognitive behavioral condition reported greater decreases in solicitous responses to their child's symptoms compared to parents in the comparison condition. Figure 2-2 illustrates this finding for child pain.[4]

Turning to the second question then of what families can do to prevent or eliminate functional abdominal pain, it must first be recognized that functional abdominal pain, in children as well as adults, is the result of complex interactions between what is going on in

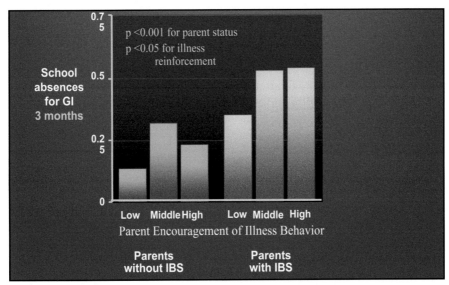

Figure 2-1. Maternal solicitousness (reinforcement) and parental IBS related to school absences. (Reprinted from Levy RL, Whitehead WE, Walker LS, et al. Increased somatic complaints and health-care utilization in children: effects of parent IBS status and parent response to gastrointestinal symptoms. *Am J Gastroenterol.* 2004;99(12):2442-2451.)

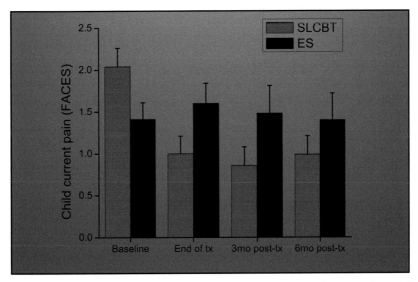

Figure 2-2. Child current pain significantly better in the experimental than control group 6 months following treatment. (Reprinted from Levy RL, Langer SL, Walker LS, et al. Cognitive-behavioral therapy for children with functional abdominal pain and their parents decreases pain and other symptoms. *Am J Gastroenterol.* 2010;105(4):946-956.)

the body and how the mind responds to what is going on in the body. Clearly, physicians must first thoroughly determine if factors such as lactose intolerance, other allergies, or other biologic factors are the cause of a child's symptoms and if a simple solution is available. Once easy first steps have been taken, the suggestions below provide some important steps that can be taken to reduce the impact of functional abdominal pain:

- As with adult IBS, education and reassurance to parents and children is the best first step. This alone may reduce both parent and child distress, which has been shown to exacerbate symptoms.

- Parental response to children's complaints should be explored. Parents should be supported to model *and encourage* wellness, rather than to support inappropriate illness behaviors in their children.

- If it is determined that significant levels of parent and/or child psychological distress exist or if there are unhelpful interactions between parents and children that are beyond the level that can be addressed in the physician's office, referral to a competent mental health professional should be considered.

Summary

Functional abdominal pain of childhood appears to be related to both physical and social learning processes. Many children appear to learn a way of responding to their physiological sensations in general from their parents in a way that adversely affects their ability to cope with these sensations. Using this information, physicians working with parents, children, and sometimes mental health professionals can have a significant impact on this disabling problem.

References

1. Levy RL, Jones KR, Whitehead WE, Feld SI, Talley NJ, Corey LA. Irritable bowel syndrome in twins: heredity and social learning both contribute to etiology. *Gastroenterology.* 2001;121(4):799-804.
2. Mulvaney S, Lambert EW, Garber J, Walker LS. Trajectories of symptoms and impairment for pediatric patients with functional abdominal pain: a 5-year longitudinal study. *J Am Acad Child Adolesc Psych.* 2006;45(6):737-744.
3. Levy RL, Whitehead WE, Walker LW, et al. Increased somatic complaints and health care utilization in children: effects of parent IBS status and parent response to gastrointestinal symptoms. *Am J Gastroenterol.* 2004;99:2442-2451.
4. Levy RL, Langer SL, Walker LS, et al. Cognitive-behavioral therapy for children with functional abdominal pain and their parents decreases pain and other symptoms. *Am J Gastroenterol.* 2010;105:946-956.

WHAT IS THE NATURAL HISTORY OF IBS?

Larissa Fujii, MD; Lucinda A. Harris, MD; and
Michael D. Crowell, PhD, FACG, AGAF

Irritable bowel syndrome (IBS) is characterized by chronic episodic abdominal pain or discomfort that is associated with relapsing and remitting constipation and/or diarrhea. The most recent diagnostic criteria proposed by the Rome III international working group on functional gastrointestinal disorders (shown in Table 3-1) proposed that patients be classified based on stool characteristics as IBS with constipation (IBS-C), IBS with diarrhea (IBS-D), IBS mixed type (IBS-M), and IBS unsubtyped (IBS-U).

IBS is a prevalent condition with 7% to 10% of the population estimated to have the disorder worldwide. The onset of symptoms generally occurs in early adulthood and has a female predominance of approximately twice that of males. However, it has recently been recognized as a component of Gulf War Syndrome, a multi-symptom complex affecting soldiers (predominantly male) from the Persian Gulf War. The prevalence of IBS among Caucasians, African Americans, and Hispanics appears to be very similar. Although most IBS patients do not seek medical attention, healthcare visits related to IBS still represent a substantial portion of visits to primary-care providers and gastroenterologists, accounting for approximately 12% of primary-care clinic visits and up to 28% of gastroenterology visits in the United States. IBS sufferers experience a threefold increase in absences from work and undergo more frequent medical testing and abdominal surgery than do non-IBS patients. As a consequence, considerable costs, both direct and indirect, are associated with IBS.

Because IBS has been considered a "diagnosis of exclusion," there may be concern that significant gastrointestinal disease may have been overlooked. However, it has been shown that a symptom-based diagnostic approach (eg, Rome criteria presented in Table 3-2), together with a thorough history and physical examination to assess for alarm symptoms and selected tests to exclude organic disease is effective and rarely results in missed IBS diagnoses. The presence of alarm symptoms, however, should prompt

---

Table 3-1

Subtypes of IBS by Predominant Stool Pattern

- IBS-C
  IBS with Constipation, defined as hard or lumpy stools ≥ 25% and loose (mushy) or watery stools < 25% of bowel movements, in the absence of antidiarrheals or laxatives
- IBS-D
  IBS with diarrhea, defined as loose (mushy) or watery stools ≥ 25% and hard or lumpy stool < 25% of bowel movements, in the absence of antidiarrheals or laxatives
- IBS-M
  Mixed IBS, defined as hard or lumpy stools ≥ 25% and loose (mushy) or watery stools ≥ 25% of bowel movements, in the absence of antidiarrheals or laxatives
- IBS-Unsubtyped
  Insufficient abnormality of stool consistency to meet criteria for IBS-C, D, or M

Table 3-2

Diagnosis of IBS

*The Rome III Diagnostic Criteria**
*Recurrent abdominal pain or discomfort** at least 3 days per month in the last 3 months associated with 2 or more of the following:* 1) Improvement with defecation 2) Onset associated with a change in frequency of stool 3) Onset associated with a change in form (appearance) of stool
Other symptoms that are not essential but support the diagnosis of IBS: • Abnormal stool frequency (greater than 3 bowel movements/day or less than 3 bowel movements/week); • Abnormal stool form (lumpy/hard or loose/watery stool); • Abnormal stool passage (straining, urgency, or feeling of incomplete bowel movement); • Passage of mucus; • Bloating or feeling of abdominal distension.

*Criteria fulfilled for the last 3 months with symptom onset at least 6 months prior to diagnosis.
**"Discomfort" means an uncomfortable sensation not described as pain.

---

further investigation (Table 3-3). A sample diagnostic algorithm is presented in Figure 3-1. Screening tests such as complete blood count, serum chemistries, and thyroid function tests are not helpful in establishing the diagnosis of IBS. The prevalence of structural abnormalities of the colon has been shown to be no higher in IBS patients than in healthy

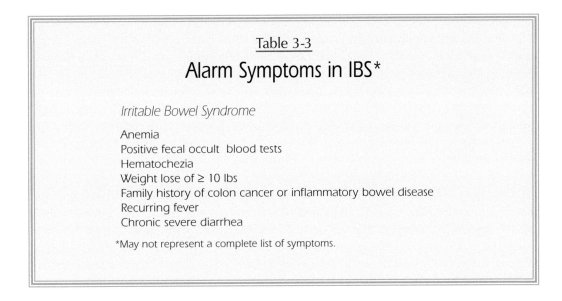

Table 3-3

Alarm Symptoms in IBS*

Irritable Bowel Syndrome

Anemia
Positive fecal occult blood tests
Hematochezia
Weight lose of ≥ 10 lbs
Family history of colon cancer or inflammatory bowel disease
Recurring fever
Chronic severe diarrhea

*May not represent a complete list of symptoms.

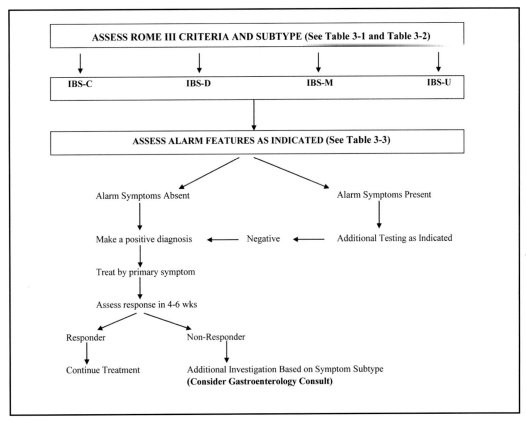

Figure 3-1. Assess Rome III criteria and subtype.

controls,[1] although in patients with IBS-D, recent American College of Gastroenterology (ACG) guidelines support random colon biopsies to rule out microscopic colitis. Celiac disease is another exception because it presents with symptoms that mimic IBS, such as bloating, diarrhea, and abdominal pain. In addition, the prevalence of celiac disease in the Western world is greater than 1%, and recent studies demonstrate that the prevalence is higher among patients with IBS than the general population. Therefore, current ACG guidelines advocate routine celiac disease serology in patients with IBS-D or IBS-M.[2]

Symptoms of IBS may fluctuate between constipation and diarrhea subtypes, and overlap with other functional GI disorders, such as functional dyspepsia, is common. In one prospective study of patients over 3 months, approximately half of patients with IBS-D or IBS-C were found to switch to alternating symptoms of diarrhea and constipation.[3] Pain-predominant and IBS-M patients were more stable with little change in their predominant symptoms. Gender also may play a role in IBS symptoms and the course of the disease. Although GI symptoms have been shown to be common in women during the menstrual cycle, women with IBS reported more intense symptoms during the late luteal phase and early menses phase. Oral contraceptives have been shown to improve dysmenorrhea symptoms, but their effect on GI symptoms has not been demonstrated. Women with IBS have also been shown to be more likely to have abdominal surgeries, and some women have reported the onset of GI symptoms after gynecological surgery.[4]

A variety of nongastrointestinal somatic complaints, such as chronic fatigue, myalgia, sleep disturbance, headache, dysuria, and sexual dysfunction, frequently co-exist in IBS patients. Consequently, IBS is frequently associated with co-morbid conditions such as fibromyalgia, chronic fatigue syndrome, interstitial cystitis, migraine headaches, and other pain syndromes. Anxiety and depression occur more commonly in IBS patients, particularly as the severity of symptoms worsens. As a result of the gastrointestinal and nongastrointestinal symptoms and psychological co-morbidities, impaired quality of life in IBS patients is common. Patients with IBS have an increased risk of suicide that is two to four times higher than those individuals without IBS symptoms. This increased risk may be attributable to the increased prevalence of psychological disturbances, poor quality of life, inadequate therapy, maladaptive coping mechanisms to stressors, and patients' negative emotions.[5] Depression, ineffective coping, substance abuse, co-morbidities such as insomnia and fibromyalgia, and length and severity of symptoms have also been found to be risk factors for suicidal ideation. Finally, a history of abuse, sexual and/or physical, has been associated with severe symptoms of IBS and may influence treatment choices and the course of the disease.

Overall, the prognosis of IBS is good, and few studies have demonstrated significant morbidity or mortality over the long term in IBS patients. Once made, the diagnosis of IBS is reasonably stable with only about one-third of patients achieving complete resolution of their symptoms at a median follow-up of 2 years.[6] Patients typically have exacerbations of their symptoms followed by periods of remission. In one study, 30% of IBS patients reported resolution of symptoms at 1 year, but only 5% remained symptom-free after 5 years.[7] In another study that followed the clinical course of patients over 3 months, it was observed that most patients had symptoms for more than 50% of the days and on average had 12.4 episodes of recurrent symptoms. However, the duration of exacerbations was relatively short, averaging only about 5 days.[8] Positive prognostic factors for symptom remission include constipation-predominant subtype, brief history (less than 2 years) of symptoms, presentation with diarrhea, and postinfectious IBS.[9] Poor prognostic factors include psychological co-morbidities, especially anxiety, and those with previous abdominal surgeries.

Summary

IBS is a common chronic disorder that is associated with considerable disability and cost. A symptom-based diagnostic approach with selected tests to exclude organic disease is effective and rarely results in missed diagnoses, but the presence of alarm symptoms should prompt further investigation. Limited testing, including evaluation for celiac disease in patients with IBS-D and IBS-M, is recommended. Symptom intensity and bowel alterations fluctuate between constipation and diarrhea subtypes and overlap with other functional GI disorders. Gender influences the course of the disease, and women with IBS report intensification of symptoms during menses. Symptom fluctuation in males has not been well established. Gastrointestinal symptoms and psychological co-morbidities result in impaired quality of life in IBS patients. Although significant morbidity and mortality over the long-term in IBS patients is rare, these patients do have an increased risk of suicide. Overall, the prognosis of IBS is good, and symptoms may improve over time, but they rarely resolve completely without intervention.

References

1. Chey WD, Nojkov B, Rubenstein JH, Dobhan RR, Greenson JK, Cash BD. The yield of colonoscopy in patients with non-constipated irritable bowel syndrome: Results from a prospective, controlled US trial. *Am J Gastroenterol.* 2010;105(4):859-865.
2. Brandt LJ, Chey WD, Foxx-Orenstein AE, et al. An evidence-based systematic review on the management of irritable bowel syndrome—American College of Gastroenterology task force on IBS. *Am J Gastroenterol.* 2009;104:S1-S35.
3. Mearin F, Baro E, Roset M, Badia X, Zarate N, Perez I. Clinical patterns over time in irritable bowel syndrome: symptom instability and severity variability. *Am J Gastroenterol.* 2004;99(1):113-121.
4. Heitkemper M, Jarrett M. Irritable bowel syndrome; does gender matter? *J Psychosom Res.* 2008;64(6): 583-587.
5. Spiegel B, Schoenfeld P, Naliboff B. Systematic review: the prevalence of suicidal behavior in patients with chronic abdominal pain and irritable bowel syndrome. *Aliment Pharmacol Ther.* 2007;26(2):183-193.
6. El-Serag HB, Pilgrim P, Schoenfeld P. Systematic review: natural history of irritable bowel syndrome. *Aliment Pharmacol Ther.* 2004;19:861-870.
7. Cremonini F, Talley NJ. Irritable bowel syndrome: epidemiology, natural history, health care seeking, and emerging risk factors. *Gastroenterol Clin North Am.* 2005;34:189-204.
8. Hahn B, Watson M, Yan S, Gunput D, Heuijerjans J. Irritable bowel syndrome symptom patterns: frequency, duration, and severity. *Dig Dis Sci.* 1998;43:2715-2718.
9. Janssen HAM, Muris JWM, Knotterus JA. The clinical course and prognostic determinants of the irritable bowel syndrome: a literature review. *Scand J Gastroenterol.* 1998;33:561-567.

SECTION II

DIAGNOSIS AND PATIENT IMPACT

How Can I Diagnose IBS?

Nicholas J. Talley, MD, PhD, FACP, FRACP, FRCP, and
Steven J. Bollipo, MBBS, FRACP

In the past, irritable bowel syndrome (IBS) was considered a diagnosis of exclusion, but this has changed. A confident diagnosis of IBS can and should be made in clinical practice, but there are caveats—some patients will need at least minimal investigations to confirm the clinical impression, and, in those with atypical presentations, careful consideration of the differential diagnosis is important. We will describe here our approach to diagnosis and the evidence supporting it; despite being a common condition, there are several myths regarding the diagnosis of IBS that will be exposed.

Step 1. Take the History!

You should suspect IBS in any patient who presents with a history of abdominal pain (or discomfort) *and* disturbed defecation (diarrhea, constipation, or mixed pattern) for 3 months or longer. The pain is directly related to bowel dysfunction, usually waxes and wanes (and is virtually never continuous), can occur in the lower abdomen or at any abdominal site, may be precipitated by eating, and is not usually induced by menstruation, urination, or physical activity. Abdominal bloating is also very common, and some patients note visible distension; some experts argue the absence of bloating should lead one to question a diagnosis of IBS, but bloating is not required for diagnosis.[1] Ask patients exactly what they mean if constipation or diarrhea is reported; in IBS, the stool pattern is classically irregular. Many patients with IBS also will report nausea or extraintestinal symptoms, such as fatigue, anxiety, or depression. A firm diagnosis of IBS actually relies on you asking some very simple questions that should be routine.[2]

After establishing the details of the pain, bowel disturbance, and bloating, ask the patient the following questions:

1. Is your pain (or discomfort) relieved by defecation?
2. At the onset of the pain, are your stools looser or harder?
3. At the onset of the pain, do you have more (or less) frequent stools?

If the answer is yes to 2 or more of these questions, your patient likely fulfills the Rome III criteria for IBS. A number of different sets of diagnostic criteria (Tables 4-1 and 4-2) evolved into the current Rome III criteria.[2] The Rome I, Manning, and Kruis criteria have all been formally validated. The Rome II and III criteria were derived from these; although the most recent criteria (Rome III) are also the most widely used, they are yet to be validated.[3] However, they appear to function perfectly well in practice.

Next, try to establish if he or she has diarrhea-predominant, constipation-predominant, or mixed IBS based on the stool form (Table 4-3). Patients can find it difficult or even embarrassing to describe the appearance of stool. In practice, the best way to obtain a consistent description of stool form is to use the Bristol Stool Chart.[4]

What should you do if the patient does *not* fulfill Rome criteria? Remember, the Rome criteria are specific but not sensitive; the absence of the criteria does *not* mean the patient doesn't have IBS. Asking the 6 Manning symptom criteria can help (see Table 4-2); the presence of 3 or more of these symptoms is strongly suggestive of IBS, too. The American College of Gastroenterology IBS Task Force[5] has recommended a simpler definition for IBS than Rome (abdominal pain or discomfort associated with altered bowel habits over a period of at least 3 months), but this definition, while sensitive, appears not to be very specific. Hence, if a patient fails to fulfill Rome or Manning criteria but you suspect IBS, you need to undertake a more detailed clinical evaluation to try and exclude other causes before concluding the diagnosis is IBS (see Table 4-4).

Abdominal pain and altered bowel habits can be caused by many other conditions including small bowel bacterial overgrowth, lactose intolerance, celiac sprue, inflammatory bowel disease, and, importantly, colorectal cancer. Sometimes out of fear of missing a serious diagnosis, physicians will routinely order a battery of investigations before committing the patient to a diagnosis of IBS, but this is neither economical nor clinically appropriate.[6]

Step 2. Look for Red Flags (Alarm Features)

To help clinch the diagnosis, specifically probe the patient for any alarm symptoms, which should all be absent (Table 4-5). Then, you need to do a complete physical examination to make sure there are no alarm signs. Do not confuse abdominal wall pain (increases with tensing the abdominal wall muscles) with deep tenderness sometimes found in IBS.

If the patient answers yes to any of these alarm symptom questions or has an alarm sign, you need to be concerned that there may be an alternative diagnosis (eg, weight loss and gastrointestinal cancer; vomiting and small bowel obstruction; blood loss and inflammatory bowel disease). Remember, red flags raise the pre-test probability that there is underlying structural disease, but most patients with one alarm feature will not be found during subsequent evaluation to have a serious organic explanation for their symptoms.[7] The investigation of alarm features depends on the findings; often, a colonoscopy is the first test considered. In the United States, all patients 50 years and older are routinely offered a colonoscopy (if not previously performed) or an alternative test to screen for colon cancer; age is thus an alarm feature, and colon cancer screening recommendations apply to those with and without suspected IBS (although, remember that finding polyps or even an incidental cancer in the setting of suspected IBS usually means the patient has IBS plus the colonic pathology).

Table 4-1

Comparing Proposed Diagnostic Criteria for the Diagnosis of Irritable Bowel Syndrome

Criteria or Model	Kruis et al, 1984	Rome I, 1990	Rome II, 1999	Rome III, 2006
Symptoms	Symptoms reported by the patient: Abdominal pain, flatulence, or bowel irregularity. Description of abdominal pain as "burning, cutting, very strong, terrible, feeling of pressure, dull, boring, or 'not so bad'"	Abdominal pain or discomfort relieved with defecation or associated with a change in stool frequency or consistency, plus >2 of the following on at least 25% of occasions or days: Altered stool frequency; Altered stool form; Altered stool passage; Passage of mucus per rectum; Bloating or distension	Abdominal discomfort or pain that has two of three features: Relieved with defecation; Onset associated with a change in frequency of stool; Onset associated with a change in form of stool	Recurrent abdominal pain or discomfort >3 days per month in the last 3 months associated with two or more of the following: Improvement with defecation; Onset associated with a change in frequency of stool; Onset associated with a change in form of stool
Signs	As determined by a physician: Abnormal physical findings and/or history pathognomonic for any diagnosis other than IBS			
Laboratory investigations	ESR>20 mm/2 h Leukocytosis >10,000 cells/microliter; Anemia (Hemoglobin <12 g/dL for women or <14 g/dL for men); Blood in the stools			
Symptom duration required	>2 years	>3 months	>12 weeks (need not be consecutive) in the last 1 year	Symptom onset >6 months prior to diagnosis

Table 4-2
Manning Criteria

1. Abdominal pain relieved by defecation

2. More frequent stools with onset of pain

3. Looser stools with onset of pain

4. Passage of mucus per rectum

5. Feeling of incomplete rectal emptying

6. Patient-reported visible abdominal distension

Table 4-3
IBS Types by Stool Form

1. IBS with constipation (IBS-C)	Hard or lumpy stools >25% of the time (with loose [mushy] or watery stools <25% of bowel movements)
2. IBS with diarrhea (IBS-D)	Loose (mushy) or watery stools >25% of the time (and hard or lumpy stools <25% of bowel movements)
3. Mixed IBS (IBS-M)	Hard or lumpy stools >25% and loose (mushy) or watery stools >25% of bowel movements
4. Unsubtyped IBS	Insufficient abnormality of stool consistency to meet criteria for IBS-C, -D, or -M.

Step 3. Targeted Investigations

If the patient fulfills Rome or Manning criteria and has no alarm features, one can be reasonably confident the diagnosis is IBS (Figure 4-1); we advise you to make a positive diagnosis and to inform the patient at the first visit. A positive diagnosis is reassuring and reduces health-care seeking behavior in IBS.[8] However, you will still need to order testing in selected settings; we recommend counseling the patient that this is being done to rule out other very uncommon explanations and the yield is low.

Testing recommended by the ACG Taskforce depends on the IBS subgroup:

1. **If diarrhea or a mixed bowel pattern is present, testing for celiac disease serologically is recommended (eg, tissue transglutaminase—tTG).** The prevalence

Table 4-4

Differential Diagnosis of Irritable Bowel Syndrome

Differential Diagnosis	*Clinical Clues*	*Diagnostic Tests*
Small intestinal bacterial overgrowth (SIBO)	Previous abdominal surgery Bloating and diarrhea in diabetes mellitus or scleroderma	Lactulose breath test Glucose breath test Quantitative duodenal aspirate culture Trial of antibiotic therapy
Lactose intolerance	Diarrhea, abdominal pain and flatulence after ingestion of milk or milk-containing products	Trial of lactose-free diet Lactose breath test
Celiac disease	Diarrhea, weight loss, anemia, iron deficiency, gluten intolerance	Serology for celiac antibodies (t-TG antibodies) Duodenal biopsy
Inflammatory bowel disease (Crohn's and ulcerative colitis)	Nocturnal symptoms, weight loss, blood and mucus in the stools, anemia	Colonoscopy Small bowel capsule study
Infectious diarrhea (eg, Giardia, parasites in endemic areas)	History of travel, history of exposure	Stool microscopy, culture
Colon cancer	Family history of colon cancer, rectal bleeding, weight loss, recent change in bowel habits in patients older than 50 years	Colonoscopy

of celiac disease is increased in those presenting with IBS symptoms (about 5% are so affected).[9] If serology is positive, the patient deserves a small bowel biopsy to confirm the diagnosis of sprue. Rarely, constipation can be a presenting symptom of sprue.

2. **If constipation is the predominant bowel pattern, no testing is routinely required.** However, we suggest considering anorectal manometry and balloon expulsion testing to rule out pelvic floor dysfunction if standard treatment for constipation fails. It is our experience that many IBS patients also have paradoxical anal sphincter contraction on straining that is a major contributor to their constipation.

3. **Other tests.** No other tests are routinely recommended but a selected few may be considered if symptoms are severe or atypical or if they fail to respond to standard therapy. Stool microscopy can occasionally be useful to exclude infections such as Giardia and other parasites in endemic areas. The presence of leukocytes in the stool

Table 4-5

Alarm Features That Should Alert You to the Possibility of Other Diagnoses

Alarm Features	Possible Diagnosis	Tests Recommended
Rectal bleeding	Colon cancer, inflammatory bowel disease	Colonoscopy
Weight loss	Colon cancer, celiac disease, other malabsorption syndromes	Upper endoscopy, duodenal biopsy, colonoscopy
Vomiting	Bowel obstruction	Cross-sectional abdominal imaging
Anemia or iron deficiency	Celiac disease, colon cancer, inflammatory bowel disease	Upper endoscopy, duodenal biopsy, colonoscopy
Family history of other GI conditions	Colon cancer, inflammatory bowel disease, celiac disease	Upper endoscopy, duodenal biopsy, colonoscopy, celiac serology
Fever	Diverticulitis, abscess, inflammatory bowel disease	Abdominal CT scan
Abdominal mass	Colon cancer, Crohn's disease	Abdominal CT scan
Age >50	Colon cancer	Colonoscopy

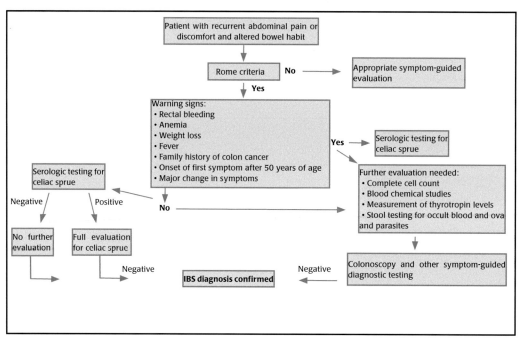

Figure 4-1. Differential diagnosis. (Reprinted with permission from Mayer EA. Clinical practice. Irritable bowel syndrome. *N Engl J Med.* 2008;358(16):1692-1699.)

should alert one to the possibility of inflammatory bowel disease or an infectious colitis. In such cases, a colonoscopy with biopsies is recommended to rule out inflammation. If there is a history of persistent watery diarrhea, colonoscopy and biopsies can exclude microscopic colitis, which can otherwise be indistinguishable from IBS.[10] Think about laxative abuse in difficult cases. Other stool tests under investigation include measuring calprotectin (to screen for inflammatory bowel disease) and serine proteases (increased in IBS) but these remain experimental.

Complete blood count, serum chemistry, and thyroid function tests have no greater yield in patients with IBS compared with the general population,[11] but if you are worried about anemia (eg, you note pallor) or find signs suggestive of thyroid disease, you should test!

To identify small intestinal bacterial overgrowth in patients with IBS and bloating, some recommend a lactulose breath test (the results of which are confounded by fast intestinal transit) or a glucose breath test (which is more specific) but the value of such testing is unclear.[12]

Lactose intolerance is more prevalent in IBS patients (38%) compared to healthy controls (20%).[13] However, the most useful test to exclude lactose intolerance (and the cheapest) is dietary modification (withdraw all lactose for 2 weeks). If lactose intolerance remains a concern despite dietary modification, lactose breath testing may be considered.

Avoid unnecessary CT scans, although occasionally CT enterography or a small bowel capsule study will identify overlooked Crohn's disease. Endometriosis can present with mid-cycle pain and often requires laparoscopy to confirm the diagnosis. Ovarian cancer is rare but can present with IBS-like symptoms in women, so a pelvic exam and ultrasound may be worthwhile if you are at all worried.

Take Home Points

Make a positive diagnosis of IBS; this approach will benefit your patients. IBS can be accurately diagnosed by careful history taking (asking focused questions), physical examination, and limited or no laboratory tests in patients with typical IBS symptoms and no alarm features. Celiac serology testing is now routine if diarrhea is present. More extensive investigations including colonoscopy should be limited to those with alarm features or those who experience a major change in clinical features during follow-up or fail to respond to standard therapy.

References

1. Houghton LA, Lea R, Agrawal A, Reilly B, Whorwell PJ. Relationship of abdominal bloating to distention in irritable bowel syndrome and effect of bowel habit. *Gastroenterology.* 2006;131(4):1003-1010.
2. Ford AC, Talley NJ, Veldhuyzen van Zanten SJ, Vakil NB, Simel DL, Moayyedi P. Will the history and physical examination help establish that irritable bowel syndrome is causing this patient's lower gastrointestinal tract symptoms? *JAMA.* 2008;300:1793-1805.
3. Jellema P, van der Windt DA, Schellevis FG, van der Horst HE. Systematic review: Accuracy of symptom based criteria for diagnosis of irritable bowel syndrome in primary care. *Aliment Pharmacol Ther.* 2009;30:695-706.
4. O'Donnell LJD, Virjee J, Heaton KW. Detection of pseudodiarrhoea by simple clinical assessment of intestinal transit rate. *Br Med J.* 1990;300:439-440.
5. American College of Gastroenterology Task Force on Irritable Bowel Syndrome, Brandt LJ, Chey WD, Foxx-Orenstein AE, Schiller LR, Schoenfeld PS, Spiegel BM, Talley NJ, Quigley EM. An evidence-based position statement on the management of irritable bowel syndrome. *Am J Gastroenterol.* 2009;104(Suppl 1): S1-S35.

6. Cash BD, Schoenfeld P, Chey WD. The utility of diagnostic tests in irritable bowel syndrome patients: a systematic review. *Am J Gastroenterol.* 2002;97:2812-2819.

7. Ford AC, Veldhuyzen van Zanten SJO, Rodgers CC, et al. Diagnostic utility of alarm features for colorectal cancer: systematic review and meta-analysis. *Gut.* 2008;57(11):1545-1553.

8. Longstreth GF, Drossman DA. Severe irritable bowel and functional abdominal pain syndromes: managing the patient and health care costs. *Clin Gastroenterol Hepatol.* 2005;3:397-400.

9. Ford AC, Chey WD, Talley NJ, Malhotra A, Spiegel BM, Moayyedi P. Yield of diagnostic tests for celiac disease in individuals with symptoms suggestive of irritable bowel syndrome. *Arch Intern Med.* 2009;169(7): 651-658.

10. Limsui D, Pardi DS, Camilleri M, et al. Symptomatic overlap between irritable bowel syndrome and microscopic colitis. *Inflamm Bowel Dis.* 2007;13(2):175-181.

11. Tolliver BA, Herrera JL, DiPalma JA. Evaluation of patients who meet clinical criteria for Irritable Bowel Syndrome. *Am J Gastroenterol.* 1994;89:176-178.

12. Bratten JR, Spanier J, Jones M. Lactulose breath testing does not discriminate patients with irritable bowel syndrome from healthy controls. *Am J Gastroenterol.* 2008;103(4):958-963.

13. Farup PG, Monsbakken KW, Vandvik PO. Lactose malabsorption in a population with irritable bowel syndrome: Prevalence and symptoms. A case control study. *Scand J Gastroenterol.* 2004;39(7):645-649.

How Do I Distinguish IBS Constipation From Other Types of Constipation?

Kalyani Meduri, MD and
Satish S. C. Rao, MD, PhD, FACG, AGAF, FRCP

Constipation and irritable bowel syndrome with constipation (IBS-C) are both chronic bowel disorders with relapsing and overlapping symptoms. They are part of a group of digestive disorders often referred to as functional gastrointestinal disorders (FGIDs). Unlike many other diseases, they are characterized by altered bowel function, hence the term functional; however, in contrast to organic disorders (ie, Crohn's disease), they lack specific biomarkers that can be measured in blood, mucosa, or stool.

Epidemiology

These two conditions affect 15% to 25% of the population. The prevalence of chronic constipation (CC) increases with age, especially in those over the age of 65 years, whereas IBS-C tends to be more common in younger individuals with a peak incidence around 40 years. CC accounts for 2.5 million physician visits annually in the United States with more than 100,000 referrals to gastroenterologists and more than $230 million in direct healthcare costs. It affects work-related productivity and leads to more absences from school. It is also associated with significantly lower quality of life and higher psychological distress. Similarly, IBS reduces quality of life, increases absenteeism at both school and work, and leads to nearly $10 billion in direct costs and much more in indirect costs.

Subtypes

In the absence of a secondary cause, such as medications, luminal obstruction, or metabolic conditions (eg, significant hypercalcemia or hypothyroidism), there are 3 main

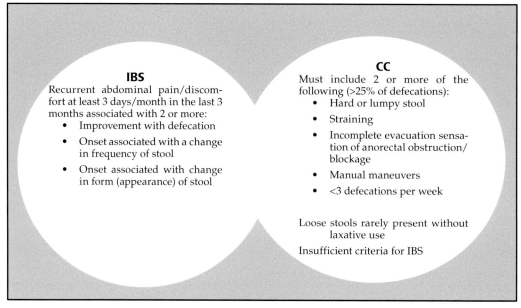

IBS
Recurrent abdominal pain/discomfort at least 3 days/month in the last 3 months associated with 2 or more:
- Improvement with defecation
- Onset associated with a change in frequency of stool
- Onset associated with change in form (appearance) of stool

CC
Must include 2 or more of the following (>25% of defecations):
- Hard or lumpy stool
- Straining
- Incomplete evacuation sensation of anorectal obstruction/blockage
- Manual maneuvers
- <3 defecations per week

Loose stools rarely present without laxative use

Insufficient criteria for IBS

Figure 5-1. Rome III diagnostic criteria of IBS and CC.

subtypes of primary constipation. However, these are not tightly compartmentalized entities, but comprise symptoms and physiologic changes that overlap in more than 50% of patients. IBS-C is characterized by abdominal pain, with or without bloating, together with altered bowel habit. These subjects may or may not have coexisting slow transit constipation or dyssynergic defecation. Slow transit and IBS-C overlap in 50% of each group.[1,2] Slow transit constipation is characterized by a prolonged delay in the transit of stool through the colon. This delay may be due to a primary dysfunction of the colonic smooth muscle (myopathy) or its nerve innervation (neuropathy), or it could be secondary to an evacuation disorder, such as dyssynergic defecation. Dyssynergic defecation, also known as obstructive defecation, anismus, pelvic floor dyssynergia, or outlet obstruction, is characterized by either difficulty or inability with expelling stool from the anorectum. Many patients with dyssynergic defecation also have prolonged colonic transit.

There is significant overlap between symptoms and the GI sensory and motility disorders that affect the upper and lower gut. About 30% of patients who present with what would typically be identified as upper GI symptoms also suffer from chronic constipation. It is important when diagnosing these disorders that this overlap is remembered and that the diagnosis of one condition does not necessarily rule out the other (Figure 5-1).[3]

Symptom Characteristics

Patients with constipation present with a broad spectrum of symptoms. Physicians recognize fewer than 3 bowel movements a week as the "typical" symptom of constipation, but it is only reported by one-third of patients with constipation. Other symptoms such as straining, hard or lumpy stools, and a feeling of incomplete emptying are of greater importance to these patients and are reported more commonly, but often are not well recognized nor inquired about by healthcare providers.

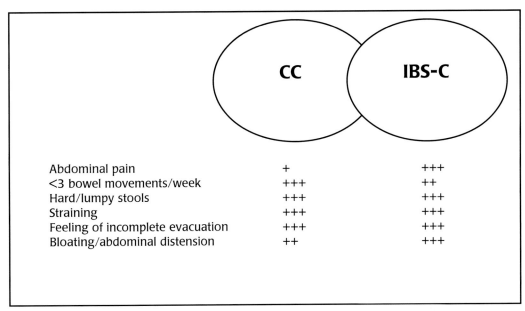

	CC	IBS-C
Abdominal pain	+	+++
<3 bowel movements/week	+++	++
Hard/lumpy stools	+++	+++
Straining	+++	+++
Feeling of incomplete evacuation	+++	+++
Bloating/abdominal distension	++	+++

Figure 5-2. Overlap of symptoms between CC and IBS-C.

Patients with IBS-C have similar symptoms to constipation, such as straining, hard or lumpy stools, decreased bowel movement frequency, and the sensation of incomplete evacuation. What differentiates IBS-C from other types of constipation is the presence of abdominal pain, with or without bloating, together with an altered bowel habit (Figure 5-2). These subjects may or may not have slow transit or dyssynergia. Patients exhibiting little or no abdominal pain are more likely to be labeled as having chronic constipation, whereas those experiencing abdominal discomfort are more likely suffering from IBS-C. Colon transit is prolonged in primary constipation whereas IBS patients have normal transit and normal anorectal manometry. Rectal sensory testing may reveal hypersensitivity in 50% to 60% of patients with IBS-C.

Crowell et al[4] compared the distribution of gastrointestinal symptoms among IBS-C patients and functional constipation patients and found a significant overlap for both lower GI and upper GI symptoms in patients with IBS-C and functional constipation. They found that the symptom complex of frequent abdominal pain, excessive intestinal gas, and the sensation of incomplete evacuation best differentiates IBS-C patients from those with functional constipation.

Diagnostic Tests

Chronic constipation and IBS are syndromes (ie, collections of symptoms). The pre-test likelihood of a diagnosis of CC or IBS in patients meeting symptom criteria (Rome III) and without alarm features is approximately 90%. The same is not true for patients with upper GI symptoms. It is important to use tests/investigations selectively and only when the results will make a difference in patient management. Serological tests for celiac disease may be considered in some patients.[5] A list of alarm features is shown in Table 5-1. A list of tests recommended for evaluating these patients is shown in Tables

Table 5-1
Alarm Features for IBS/CC[6]

- Refractory or worsening IBS symptoms or nocturnal pain
- Older patients (≥50 years old) with first presentation
- Blood in stool or guaiac-positive stool
- Anemia
- Weight loss (unintentional)
- Anorexia
- Family history of organic GI disease (celiac disease, IBD, colorectal cancer)

Table 5-2
Tests That Are Recommended for Routine Diagnostic Evaluation in Patients with IBS-C and CC and in Patients With Alarm Features

Routine Diagnostic Tests

- CBC/ESR/electrolytes/metabolic panel
- Thyroid function
- Tissue transglutaminase antibody (TTG)

Diagnostic Tests for Patients With Alarm Features

- Flexible sigmoidoscopy
- Colonoscopy
- Colon/rectal biopsy
- Barium enema
- Ultrasound scan of abdomen
- CAT scan
- Breath test and motility tests
- Stool tests

5-2 and 5-3. Some patients with symptoms consistent with functional disorders have additional symptoms and signs that may indicate an alternative diagnosis or comorbid illness. In such patients, one would consider additional diagnostic testing to identify causes for the symptoms.

Table 5-3

Specific Diagnostic Tests for Further Evaluation of Patients With Chronic Constipation and IBS-C Together With Their Clinical Significance

Constipation		IBS	
Test	Significance	Test	Significance
Colonic transit study	Evaluate slow or normal transit constipation	Rectal balloon distention/ sensation	Evaluate rectal hypersensitivity
Wireless motility capsule test	Evaluate gastric emptying, small bowel transit, colonic and whole gut transit	Glucose breath test	Evaluate bacterial overgrowth
Anorectal manometry	Evaluate dyssynergia, Rectal hyposensitivity or Rectal hypersensitivity	Fructose breath test	Dietary fructose intolerance/ malabsorption
Balloon expulsion test	Evaluate dyssynergic defecation	Lactose breath test	Dietary lactose intolerance/ malabsorption
Defecography	Evaluate pelvic floor dyssynergia		

In individuals with symptoms of constipation that are not responding to empirical therapy or laxatives, it is reasonable to consider further testing.[6] Table 5-4 provides suggestions regarding when to refer these patients for further specialist evaluation. Desperate individuals may demand surgery, and it is important that surgery be avoided as long as possible and patients dissuaded from considering this option. Many unnecessary surgeries are performed in these patients.

Summary

Although there is an overlap of symptoms and pathophysiology between IBS-C and CC, in clinical practice, it is possible to distinguish these two conditions in the vast majority of patients through a careful history and detailed characterization of their presenting symptoms and comorbid features and, if necessary, through appropriate testing.

Table 5-4

When to Refer a Patient With IBS or CC to a Specialist

- The diagnosis is in doubt
- The patient is not responding to therapy
- There is rectal bleeding, anal pain or alarm features
- Invasive procedure/further hospital-based investigations are planned
- Consideration of counseling or psychiatry
- Consideration of gastrointestinal motility tests

References

1. Rao SSC. Constipation: evaluation and treatment of colonic and anorectal motility disorders. *Gastroenterol Clin North Am.* 2007;36:687-711.
2. Mertz H, Naliboff B, Mayer E. Physiology of refractory chronic constipation. *Am J Gastroenterol.* 1999;94:609-615.
3. Longstreth GF, Thompson WG, Chey WD, Houghton LA, Mearin F, Spiller RC. Functional bowel disorders. *Gastroenterology.* 2006;130:1480-1491.
4. Crowell MD, Schattler-Duncan A, Dennis EH. Symptomatic differentiation of irritable bowel syndrome with constipation vs. functional constipation. *Am J Gastroenterol.* 2002;97:308.
5. Cash BD, Schoenfield P, Chey WD. The utility of diagnostic tests in IBS patients, a systemic review. *Am J Gastroenterol.* 2002;97:2182-2189.
6. Lembo A, Camilleri M. Chronic constipation. *N Engl J Med.* 2003;349:1360-1368.

WHAT TESTS ARE REQUIRED TO MAKE THE DIAGNOSIS OF IBS?

Madhusudan Grover, MD and Amy E. Foxx-Orenstein, DO, FACG, FACP

Irritable bowel syndrome (IBS) is characterized by the presence of recurrent abdominal pain or discomfort in association with disordered defecation. It is the most extensively studied functional gastrointestinal disorder (FGID), despite being less prevalent than functional dyspepsia (see Chapter 23). Survey studies have shown that up to 7% to 20% of adults fulfill the diagnostic criteria for IBS. Most of these patients, however, do not seek health care. That being said, the impact of IBS on our healthcare system is substantial. For example, approximately 2% of adult primary-care visits and up to 50% of gastroenterology office visits are for the evaluation of IBS symptoms. In addition, billions of dollars are lost each year in the United States due to the direct and indirect medical costs of IBS.

The Definition

The first systematic attempt to characterize IBS (then called "irritable colon syndrome" or ICS) was made by Chaudhary and Truelove in Oxford, England in 1962. In 1976, Manning and colleagues reported results from a questionnaire distributed to Bristol Wales outpatients presenting with abdominal pain and disordered bowel habit. Six of 15 symptoms were reported more commonly in IBS compared to organic bowel disease, which formed the first criteria to diagnose IBS called the *Manning criteria*. Further need for consensus guidelines for the study and management of IBS served as the inspiration for the first Rome criteria presented at the 13th International Congress of Gastroenterology in Rome in 1988. These guidelines were then followed by the Rome II (1999) and Rome III (2006) criteria.[1]

The diagnosis of IBS during the past decade has slowly shifted from that of a negative diagnosis approach ("diagnosis of exclusion") toward a positive diagnosis approach ("fulfillment of criteria in absence of alarm symptoms"). The expectation should now be to make a confident "positive" diagnosis of IBS rather than going through an exhaustive and often fruitless process of ruling out an "organic" cause. Table 6-1 lists Rome III diagnostic criteria

+---+
| Table 6-1 |
| # Rome III Criteria for Diagnosis of IBS |
| |
| Recurrent abdominal pain or discomfort* at least 3 days/month in the |
| past 3 months associated with 2 or more of the following: |
| • Improvement with defecation |
| • Onset associated with a change in frequency of stool |
| • Onset associated with a change in form (appearance) of stool |
| Criterion fulfilled for the past 3 months with symptom onset at |
| least 6 months prior to diagnosis. |
| |
| *"Discomfort" means an uncomfortable sensation not described as pain. |
+---+

for the diagnosis of IBS. The temporal association of pain with disordered defecation is characteristic of IBS. Using Rome III criteria, IBS is also differentiated from non-painful disorders of defecation (ie, functional diarrhea or functional constipation) and from abdominal pain not associated with problems of defecation (functional abdominal pain syndrome).

Clinical Features

The abdominal pain in IBS is visceral, episodic, and unpredictable. It is often poorly localized but mostly occurs in either the central or lower abdomen. The median period of pain is 3 days per month, interspersed with pain-free days. The pain is often precipitated by eating and improves or resolves with passage of a bowel movement and with fasting. The severity of pain, rather than the alteration in bowel habits, most closely correlates with the severity of IBS. Severe IBS, as is often encountered in tertiary-care centers, is characterized by more severe pain and causes a greater degree of healthcare utilization and impairment in quality of life.[2]

Bowel habits in IBS patients can be unpredictable. In any one patient, the diagnosis of IBS tends to remain stable; however, predominant bowel habit ("diarrhea" or "constipation") can change abruptly over time. Patients may report 1 or more days of severe diarrhea after days or weeks of constipation. The association with pain can also be unpredictable but most patients tend to report pain getting better with defecation. Personal definitions of "diarrhea" or "constipation" can also differ widely. For example, constipation is characterized by fewer than 3 bowel movements a week; yet, not all who feel constipated meet that definition. Patients often perceive small stool form as well as increased effort to defecate to be associated with constipation. Similarly, frequent passage of hard stools might erroneously be labeled as diarrhea. The Bristol stool form scale is an objective measure of stool consistency and correlates with colonic transit. Hence, Rome III considers stool form or consistency measures to characterize diarrhea or constipation.

Bloating (sensory or perceptual reflection of abdominal discomfort/fullness or enlargement) and distension (measurable increase in abdominal girth) is not a specific feature of IBS but is still reported in a significant number of IBS patients. A diurnal

---

Table 6-2
Red Flags before Considering Diagnosis of IBS

- Involuntary weight loss
- Nocturnal symptoms
- Family history of colon cancer
- Blood mixed with stools
- Recent antibiotic use
- Symptom onset when patient is older than 50 years

---

increase in abdominal girth is reported more commonly in IBS and constipated patients, whereas only half of those who report bloating have distension beyond the normal range. In addition to bloating, incomplete evacuation, straining or urgency, and the presence of increased passage of gas and burping are often reported by IBS patients but are not specific enough to be included in the criteria.

Reports from the Manning criteria have revealed that individual symptoms lack both sensitivity and specificity. However, combinations of individual symptoms yield more robust sensitivity and specificity, providing the rationale behind combining these symptoms together and classifying symptoms into syndromes as in Rome III criteria.

The Red Flags

These are the clinical signs and symptoms that need careful consideration before the diagnosis of IBS can be made (Table 6-2). These symptoms and signs are meant to improve the accuracy for discriminating patients with a higher likelihood of having structural disease from patients with a low probability of such disease, compared to symptom criteria alone. In a study by Vanner and colleagues, when patients with red flags (36% of otherwise eligible patients) were excluded from the analysis, the specificity of the Rome I criteria was 100% while the sensitivity was 65%. In summarizing the studies that have used this combined strategy, the meta-analysis by Jellema and colleagues showed a median specificity of 0.92 and sensitivity of 0.67, and the meta-analysis by Ford and colleagues showed a median specificity of 0.87 and a sensitivity of 0.84. Most red flag symptoms greatly overestimate the likelihood of organic disease. Whitehead and colleagues found that 84% of patients whom clinicians (80% primary care, 20% gastroenterology clinics) ultimately diagnosed as having IBS reported one or more red flags. Additional studies are needed that examine the sensitivity of individual red flags, alone and in combination, for predicting organic disease.

PRESENCE OF RED FLAGS

If one or more alarm features are present, further investigations are required.[2] Work-up can start with blood tests including complete blood count (CBC), inflammatory markers (erythrocyte sedimentation rate [ESR]/C-reactive protein [CRP]), calcium, tissue transglutaminase (tTGA), and thyroid stimulating hormone (TSH). Anemia or elevated inflammatory markers may indicate the presence of inflammatory bowel disease. In older patients, anemia can be concerning for a large colonic polyp or cancer. A positive tTG suggests celiac disease (approximately 95% sensitivity and specificity in secondary care). Thyroid abnormalities occur in IBS patients at the same prevalence as the general population (6%). Stool ova and parasite examination should be performed in patients with IBS and diarrhea symptoms. Single examination has poor sensitivity, and antigen testing is superior to microscopic examination. Hence, we recommend that three samples be submitted for analysis.

IBS symptoms can be mimicked by a number of other less common conditions. For example, rare causes, such as HIV infection, should be considered in a high-risk patient (intravenous drug abuse or unprotected sexual intercourse with multiple partners) presenting with weight loss and chronic diarrhea. A history of recent antibiotic use preceding the onset of symptoms should alert the clinician to the possibility of *Clostridium difficile* infection. Colonoscopy is indicated to exclude colon cancer or inflammatory bowel disease (IBD) when alarm symptoms are present. For a patient with diarrheal symptoms, biopsies should be performed at the time of colonoscopy even if the mucosa is macroscopically normal, as biopsies may reveal evidence of microscopic colitis. A recent study has shown slightly higher prevalence of microscopic colitis in suspected nonconstipated IBS patients undergoing colonoscopy as compared with healthy controls.[3] Terminal ileal examination should be requested if IBD is suspected. Additionally, barium small bowel follow-through or computed tomography (CT) enterography should be performed in patients with suspected small bowel IBD.

In patients with achlorhydria, "blind loops," diverticula, strictures, or small intestinal motility disorders (chronic intestinal pseudo-obstruction), a diagnosis of small intestinal bacterial overgrowth (SIBO) should be entertained. The prevalence and impact of SIBO in IBS patients is unclear, although it can cause symptoms of diarrhea and bloating. Clinical practice varies between "test and treat" versus "treat" strategy. Most community center practices use breath testing for the diagnosis of SIBO, while tertiary-care centers often perform culture of duodenal aspirates. The glucose breath hydrogen test is plagued by a poor sensitivity and specificity at 41.7% and 44.4%, respectively. Bile acid malabsorption (BAM) is also rare and is most reliably diagnosed by measuring the percent retention of Selenium[75] homocholic acid taurine at 7 days after dosing (Blood Selenium[75] Homocholic Acid Taurine [SeHCAT] test). Values less than 5% predict a good response to trial of cholestyramine. Values between 5% and 10% are also abnormal but only 50% respond to cholestyramine. If SeHCAT is unavailable, a trial of cholestyramine is a reasonable alternative.

ABSENCE OF RED FLAGS

If there are no alarm features, an exhaustive work-up is of low yield.[4] In a recent study, a lower prevalence of colorectal adenomas in patients with "suspected" nonconstipated IBS was seen as compared to controls. Initiating an extensive and often repetitive work-up can reflect a physician's lack of confidence and reinforce a patient's belief that something is "being missed."[4] The American College of Gastroenterology does recommend serological testing for celiac disease, especially in patients with diarrhea or mixed IBS. Also, in the presence of anemia, a cause should be fully elucidated before a diagnosis of IBS is made. CRP higher than 5 mg/L has low sensitivity (50%) but good specificity (81%) for inflammatory bowel disease and should also be measured if concomitant diarrhea and anemia are present.

Dietary Influences

IBS patients often report certain specific dietary triggers, yet elimination diets are often met with poor success. The most common exclusion diets recommended for patients involve lactose and gluten elimination. Symptoms of lactose intolerance include abdominal pain, flatulence, and diarrhea. The effects of lactose are dose related (>240 mL of milk or its equivalent). Unfortunately, there is poor correlation between reported lactose intolerance and objective lactose malabsorption. Overall, the incidence of lactose intolerance in IBS patients is similar to that of healthy people. We do not recommend lactose elimination unless it can be objectively proven as it might potentially deprive patients of an important source of calcium. A high degree of suspicion should, however, be maintained for Asians and Eastern Mediterraneans, who have a higher prevalence of lactose intolerance. It is important to also consider the potential role of fructose and related substances. There has been a recent substantial increase in ingestion of fructose, particularly in soft drinks. As fructose is poorly absorbed, large amounts can overwhelm the absorptive capacity of the small intestine leading to flatulence and diarrhea. We recommend lactose and fructose breath tests in the appropriate clinical scenario, as elimination diets in the correct clinical context can result in long-term improvements.

Summary

IBS is a common GI disorder and has significant implications in terms of quality of life, healthcare costs, and work productivity. Traditional thinking drags clinicians toward it being a diagnosis of exclusion, and an exhaustive work-up to rule out "organic" etiology is thus undertaken. Using the Rome III criteria, performing a thorough history and physical examination and ruling out "red flags" enables the clinician to confidently make a diagnosis of IBS. As discussed above, the presence of red flags warrants an appropriate evaluation. A confident positive diagnosis can be cost effective and satisfying and can lead to a therapeutic physician-patient relationship.

References

1. Longstreth GF, Thompson WG, Chey WD, Houghton LA, Mearin F, Spiller RC. Functional bowel disorders. *Gastroenterology.* 2006;130:1480-1491.
2. Spiller RC, Thompson WG. Bowel disorders. *Am J Gastroenterol.* 2010;105:775-785.
3. Chey WD, Nojkov B, Rubenstein JH, Dobhan RR, Greenson JK, Cash BD. The yield of colonoscopy in patients with non-constipated irritable bowel syndrome: results from a prospective, controlled US trial. *Am J Gastroenterol.* 2010;105:859-865.
4. Whitehead WE, Drossman DA. Validation of symptom-based diagnostic criteria for irritable bowel syndrome: a critical review. *Am J Gastroenterol.* 2010;105:814-820; quiz 813, 821.

What Is the Value of Performing a Colonoscopy in Patients With IBS?

Brooks D. Cash, MD, FACP, FACG, AGAF

The lack of reliable biomarkers and overlap of irritable bowel syndrome (IBS) symptoms with other organic conditions causes most healthcare providers to consider IBS a "diagnosis of exclusion." Because of concerns about mislabeling a patient with an organic disease with IBS, healthcare providers often order a battery of tests in patients with suspected IBS. Physicians are particularly concerned about missing colorectal cancer (CRC) or inflammatory bowel diseases (IBD), such as ulcerative colitis or Crohn's disease, in patients with IBS symptoms. Because of this, patients with typical IBS symptoms commonly undergo colonoscopy. For example, community-based surveys indicate that up to 50% of IBS patients undergo colonoscopy in the course of their diagnostic evaluation.[1] Available data suggest that 25% of all colonoscopies performed in the United States are for IBS-related symptoms and 10% of colonoscopies performed on patients younger than age 50 are conducted for evaluation of IBS symptoms. Despite such broad use of colonoscopy in the evaluation of IBS symptoms, data addressing the actual prevalence of colonic structural abnormalities in patients with IBS are limited.

In a post-hoc analysis of data from 2 placebo-controlled IBS trials, Hamm examined the yield of flexible sigmoidoscopy in study participants younger than 50 years of age or colonoscopy/flexible sigmoidoscopy and barium enema in enrollees 50 years of age or older.[2] Three hundred and six of 1452 (21%) study participants were included in this analysis, and colonic imaging identified important structural lesions in four patients (1.3%, three IBD, one colonic obstruction). Unfortunately, the results of this analysis are difficult to interpret as the proportion of patients who underwent sigmoidoscopy versus colonoscopy was not reported. Additionally, patients only underwent colonic imaging if they had not undergone such imaging within 2 years of study enrollment. Finally, the proportion of IBS patients who had undergone previous colonic imaging was not reported.

Tolliver evaluated the yield of sigmoidoscopy and barium enema and/or colonoscopy in an uncontrolled, prospective trial that included 196 subjects with suspected IBS.[3] Forty-three colonic structural abnormalities were found in 34 subjects. Most abnormalities that were identified were felt to be incidental and not responsible for patients' GI symptoms (benign polyps, diverticulosis, hemorrhoids, lipomata, and melanosis coli). Two (1.0%) patients were found to have abnormalities (one IBD, one cancer) that could have explained their IBS symptoms. Again, there are several issues that complicate interpretation of the results from this study, including the inclusion of patients with warning signs (family history of colon cancer and hemoccult positive stool), the absence of a control group, and the failure to report the percentage of IBS patients who underwent each type of examination.

In an uncontrolled study, Francis and colleagues studied the yield of flexible sigmoidoscopy, barium enema, or colonoscopy in 125 patients who fulfilled the Rome I criteria for IBS.[4] With the exception of diverticulosis, judged to be an incidental finding, no structural lesions were identified that changed the diagnosis of IBS.

Vanner performed a prospective study in 95 patients referred to gastroenterology clinics over a 9-month period in 1995–1996 who met the Rome criteria without evidence of warning signs.[5] Ninety-one percent of patients over 45 years of age underwent barium enema or colonoscopy. Two patients declined investigation, and one patient had a flexible sigmoidoscopy. Sigmoidoscopy alone was carried out in 21% of patients younger than 45 years of age. One patient with rectal bleeding was found to have ulcerative proctitis. Otherwise, no colonic abnormalities were identified.

Our group recently published the results of a study that represents the largest prospective, controlled evaluation of the diagnostic yield of colonoscopy and mucosal biopsy in patients with IBS performed to date.[6] In this cohort of patients with symptoms consistent with IBS-M or IBS-D (without warning signs), colonoscopy did not affect the diagnosis of IBS in 457 of 466 (98.1%). Structural lesions of the colon, including adenomatous and hyperplastic polyps, colorectal cancer, angiodysplasia, diverticulosis, hemorrhoids, and anal fissure, were found to be no more likely in IBS patients versus controls. Of the 1.9% of patients with suspected IBS whose diagnosis was altered as a result of performing a colonoscopy with biopsies, seven had microscopic colitis, one had Crohn's disease, and one had ulcerative colitis. Careful review of the medical records of the seven patients diagnosed with microscopic colitis indicated that they all qualified for the diagnosis of IBS-D by the Rome II criteria. If one accepts the available literature, which states that 30% to 50% of the overall IBS population falls into the IBS-M subgroup,[7] the prevalence of microscopic colitis in our study was almost certainly higher than 1.5% in those with symptoms suggestive of IBS-D. The optimal number and location of colonic mucosal biopsies needed to diagnose microscopic colitis remains controversial, so it is possible that we underestimated the true prevalence of microscopic colitis in IBS patients, as the protocol required the endoscopist to obtain only two biopsies from the sigmoid and rectum. A recent review on this topic suggested that between 18% and 34% of patients with collagenous colitis may not be identified if only rectosigmoid biopsies are obtained.[8]

Other studies have found that microscopic colitis can be mistakenly diagnosed as IBS.[9,10] These retrospective cohort analyses found that a variable proportion of patients with microscopic colitis report abdominal pain or discomfort in addition to diarrhea-related complaints. For example, Limsui and colleagues found that 56% of 131 patients from Olmstead County, Minn., diagnosed with microscopic colitis fulfilled the Rome II criteria for IBS and that 33% had been labeled as suffering with IBS prior to the diagnosis of microscopic colitis.[9] A recent retrospective analysis from the Kaiser Permanente Group in Los Angeles found that 43 of 376 (11%) patients with lymphocytic colitis and 30 of

171 (18%) patients with collagenous colitis had been labeled as suffering from IBS prior to receiving the diagnosis of microscopic colitis.[10]

Summary

The prevalence of structural abnormalities of the colon, such as polyps, colorectal cancer, and diverticulosis, appears to be no higher in patients with suspected IBS compared to healthy controls. Multiple studies evaluating the yield of lower endoscopy or imaging in patients with suspected IBS have found that fewer than 1% of these patients have IBD. A small proportion of patients with symptoms suggestive of non-constipated IBS were found to have microscopic colitis, and the likelihood of identifying microscopic colitis appears to be greater in patients with symptoms of IBS-D after age 35. The findings from these studies lend support to the recent recommendations of the American College of Gastroenterology Task Force, which state, "routine colonic imaging is not recommended in patients younger than 50 years of age with typical IBS symptoms and no alarm features. Colonoscopic imaging should be performed in IBS patients with alarm features to rule out organic diseases and in those over the age of 50 years for the purpose of colorectal cancer screening. When colonoscopy is performed in patients with IBS-D, obtaining random biopsies should be considered to rule out microscopic colitis."[11]

References

1. Talley NJ, Gabriel SE, Harmsen WS, et al. Medical costs in community subjects with irritable bowel syndrome. *Gastroenterology.* 1995;109:1736-1741.
2. Hamm LR, Sorrells SC, Harding JP, et al. Additional investigations fail to alter the diagnosis of irritable bowel syndrome in subjects fulfilling the Rome criteria. *Am J Gastroenterol.* 1999;94:1279-1282.
3. Tolliver BA, Herrera JL, DiPalma JA. Evaluation of patients who meet clinical criteria for irritable bowel syndrome. *Am J Gastroenterol.* 1994;89:176-178.
4. Francis CY, Duffy JN, Whorwell PJ, et al. Does routine abdominal ultrasound enhance diagnostic accuracy in irritable bowel syndrome? *Am J Gastroenterol.* 1996;91:1348-1350.
5. Vanner SJ, Depew WT, Paterson WG, et al. Predictive value of the Rome criteria for diagnosing the Irritable Bowel Syndrome. *Am J Gastroenterol.* 1999;94:2912-2917.
6. Chey WD, Nojkov B, Rubenstein JH, et al. The yield of colonoscopy in patients with non-constipated irritable bowel syndrome: results from a prospective, controlled US trial. *Am J Gastroenterol.* 2010;105(4):859-865.
7. Mearin F, Baro E, Roset M, et al. Clinical patterns over time in irritable bowel syndrome: Symptom instability and severity variability. *Am J Gastroenterol.* 2004;99:113-121.
8. Yantiss R, Odze R. Optimal approach to obtaining mucosal biopsies for assessment of inflammatory disorders of the gastrointestinal tract. *Am J Gastroenterol.* 2009;104:774-783.
9. Limsui D, Pardi DS, Camilleri M, et al. Symptomatic overlap between irritable bowel syndrome and microscopic colitis. *Inflammatory Bowel Diseases.* 2007;13:175-181.
10. Kao K-T, Pedraza B-A, McClune A-C, et al. Microscopic colitis: a large retrospective analysis from a health maintenance organization experience. *World J Gastroenterol.* 2009;15:3122-3127.
11. American College of Gastroenterology Task Force on Irritable Bowel Syndrome. An evidence-based position statement on the management of irritable bowel syndrome. *Am J Gastroenterol.* 2009;104(Suppl 1):S1-S35.

CAN A BLOOD TEST DIAGNOSE IBS?

Vincenzo Stanghellini, MD and Giovanni Barbara, MD

As physicians and gastroenterologists, we frequently encounter cases that elude objective evidence of an organic basis of symptoms, thereby leading to the diagnosis of a "functional bowel disorder," among which irritable bowel syndrome (IBS) is the most common. These diagnoses are somewhat disappointing for us as clinicians and are clearly quite frustrating for the patient, whose expectations of finding a "true cause" for their symptoms vanquish as each diagnostic test returns "negative or normal." Nonetheless, it is clear in the minds of all of us that organic, systemic, or metabolic diseases (inflammatory bowel disease, celiac disease, thyroid dysfunction, or gastrointestinal cancer) may also be accompanied by IBS-like symptoms and that these disorders need to be carefully excluded. In this respect, one should consider alarm features and perform blood tests to exclude anemia, inflammatory diseases, and particularly celiac disease, which is fourfold more frequent in individuals fulfilling the Rome criteria for IBS than in controls (see Chapter 22).

Once secondary disorders have been excluded, the diagnosis can be safely made based on symptom features, and the diagnosis does not place the patient at a higher risk of developing an organic disorder. Accordingly, 6-year follow-up studies indicate that fewer than 5% of patients diagnosed as being affected by IBS develop an organic condition, which does not differ from the risk of the general population. Although clinical criteria (ie, Rome III criteria) have been developed to help us in formulating a positive diagnosis, they remain scarcely popular among practicing physicians, probably due to their relative complexity and inability to match the above-mentioned expectations. Symptom-based diagnoses are also hampered in everyday practice by the frequent comorbidity of IBS with digestive and extra-digestive syndromes and the great variability of type and severity of individual symptoms (see Section IV). No wonder, then, that there is a rush to identify objective biomarkers of this common disease.[1,2]

Ideally, a diagnostic test should be highly sensitive and specific, as well as reproducible, noninvasive, and reasonably priced. The interest in the development of a diagnostic test for IBS arises from recent advances in our understanding of the complex cellular and molecular mechanisms underlying the sensory and motor dysfunctions that characterize this syndrome. Specifically, important efforts have been employed to identify abnormalities in the microbiological or biochemical content of the gut and in changes in mucosal endocrine and immunological activity.[1] The abnormal interaction between the above-mentioned pathophysiological factors has been indirectly confirmed by a recent study showing that among millions of potentially involved genes expressed in colonic mucosal biopsies, only a few that are likely involved in the host-mucosal immune response to microbial pathogens turned out to be differently expressed. Notably, these "genetic markers" were able to predict IBS in 75% of patients.[3]

Blood markers offer obvious advantages over invasive tests. A number of potential candidate circulating biomarkers of IBS have been proposed. These markers are mostly related to immune function and, in particular, focus on pro-inflammatory cytokines. In general, the current evidence suggests the presence of increased levels of plasma/serum pro-inflammatory cytokines, including interleukin (IL)-1β, tumor necrosis factor (TNF)-α, IL-6, and IL-8, as well as augmented release of similar patterns of cytokines from resting or stimulated peripheral blood mononuclear cells. Interesting data suggest that, besides pro-inflammatory cytokines, the systemic immune response may be driven by the release of TH2 cytokines, including IL-5 and IL-13, by polyclonally stimulated blood T cells. TH2 cytokines are involved in the stimulation of certain types of immune activation seen in allergic disorders, such as asthma and atopic dermatitis, as well as in parasitic infections. These tests are difficult to perform, requiring cumbersome laboratory techniques, and thus are not routinely performed. These promising results have been published in articles from a few dedicated centers and thus require further confirmation. Also, their diagnostic accuracy has not been fully evaluated. Significant overlap with control subjects exists, and high levels of pro-inflammatory cytokines have been reported in pathological conditions different from IBS, including other functional GI disorders. In general, it is largely unclear whether changes in circulating inflammatory mediators reflect what actually happens in the gut or whether these changes reflect an epiphenomenon or the expression of comorbid conditions involving organs outside the gut. For example, experimental data show increased circulating levels of cytokines in patients with depression, a typical psychosocial comorbidity of IBS. In addition, the clinical and pathophysiological heterogeneity of patients with IBS suggests that "one size may not fit all." The identification of multiple biomarkers obtained from different body sites rather than the discovery of a single blood biomarker for IBS may turn out to be the price to pay for a "molecular" diagnosis of IBS. Following this line of evidence, recent studies emphasized the potential role of the expression of genes involved in the control of pro- and anti-inflammatory cytokines, changes in the expression of molecules involved in the control of epithelial tight junctions, as well as mucosal lymphocytes and mast cells and their products. Again, none of these observations, either singly or in combination, has been translated into a diagnostic test for IBS.[1]

Quite recently, a study was specifically designed and carried out to identify a blood test for IBS. A literature search led to the identification of more than 60,000 potential biomarkers. Of these, 140 were serum-based and commercially available and were evaluated in IBS patients and controls. A sophisticated computer-assisted analysis finally selected 10 biomarkers providing the best diagnostic performance, and these included IL-1β; anti-*Saccharomyces cerevisiae* antibody (ASCA IgA); growth-related oncogene-α; anti-neutrophil cytoplasmic antibody (ANCA); antibody against CBir1; TNF-like weak inducer of apoptosis; tissue inhibitor of metalloproteinase-1; antihuman tissue transglutaminase (TTG); brain-derived neurotrophic factor (BDNF); and neutrophil gelatinase-associated lipocalin (NGAL). When tested in large cohorts of patients and controls, the specificity of the test approached 90%, but the sensitivity was only 50%, with an overall accuracy of 70%. These results need to be confirmed in large, multicenter studies, before we recommend its use in everyday practice.[1]

Summary

The rapidly growing knowledge of the pathogenetic mechanisms of IBS in the recent past is paving the way to the identification of possible biomarkers of the syndrome. At present, no laboratory diagnostic test has been identified as having a diagnostic accuracy sufficient to be routinely used in clinical practice. However, this remains a promising and exciting field of research. For the time being, therefore, the diagnosis of IBS relies on the traditional tools of good clinical practice: an accurate history-taking and physical examination with a touch of culture and a good patient-physician relationship.

References

1. Barbara G, Stanghellini V. Biomarkers in IBS: when will they replace symptoms for diagnosis and management? *Gut.* 2009;58:1571-1575.
2. Clarke G, Quigley EMM, Cryan JF, Dinan TJ. Irritable bowel syndrome: towards biomarker identification. *Trends in Molecular Medicine.* 2009;15:478-489.
3. Aerssens J, Camilleri M, Talloen W, et al. Alterations in mucosal immunity identified in the colon of patients with irritable bowel syndrome. *Clin Gastroenterol Hepatol.* 2008;6:194-205.

What Prompts Patients With IBS to Seek Out Medical Care?

Gisela Ringström, RN, PhD and Magnus Simrén, MD, PhD

Irritable bowel syndrome (IBS) is a common functional gastrointestinal (GI) disorder affecting approximately 15% of the population. The characteristic symptoms, abdominal pain and/or discomfort associated with disturbed bowel habit (ie, diarrhea, constipation, or an alteration between these two), can be severe in some patients, but also mild and tolerable in other patients.[1] A substantial number of people with IBS seek health care for their symptoms and become patients, while others manage their symptoms without consulting the healthcare system at all. The reasons for this are only partly understood.[2] Many IBS patients express negative emotional experiences of living with IBS, and health-related quality of life (HRQOL) is often affected negatively. Based on our experiences from many years of treating IBS patients, we will try to give our point of view on what prompts IBS patients to seek out medical care.

Symptoms in general are what people experience as a sign of disease and are also the primary reason for healthcare seeking. However, there are differences in how different IBS patients experience their symptoms, which influence healthcare seeking. Some patients state that they are afraid that their symptoms could be caused by a serious disease. Other patients express the view that social problems and a negative impairment in daily life due to their symptoms are the major reasons for healthcare seeking. This could include difficulties at work, avoidance of social activities, and feelings of guilt toward relatives who indirectly are negatively affected by the IBS symptoms. Furthermore, for some patients, the symptoms *per se* are so distressing that they feel the need to seek out medical care. For instance, episodes of frequent diarrhea or cramping abdominal pain could be so disabling that normal life is impossible for the patient. Moreover, a substantial number of patients with IBS, especially those with diarrhea, suffer from fecal incontinence. This has been reported to be a hidden problem in many IBS patients, which should be addressed at the initial consultation, as this is a very disabling consequence of the IBS symptoms (see Chapter 27).

Besides what is mentioned above, other factors could also be determinants for healthcare seeking. Some patients state that they are not particularly concerned about their symptoms, but their relatives are worried and have pushed the patient to seek health care—"there must be something wrong with you"—which in turn has made the patient more insecure. Furthermore, sometimes different circumstances, not directly related to the GI symptoms, drive the patient to seek health care at a particular time point, even though the severity of GI symptoms is stable. This may include psychosocial issues, such as problems with relations, work, finances etc, but also the appearance of a serious disease in a relative or a friend, which worries the patient. Therefore, the healthcare provider must take a careful history that not only focuses on the GI symptoms of the patient, but also on other factors, such as psychological well-being and social factors. This includes a question regarding why the patient comes to you at this point in time, despite the fact that symptoms have been present for a long time.

The IBS population is a very heterogeneous group, which emphasizes the importance of a multi-component treatment approach for each individual patient. A move from a pure biomedical model toward a biopsychosocial model is considered appropriate in the management of IBS patients. Asking the patient about the reason why he or she is seeking care at this point and what the patient expects from the consultation is of critical importance.

The majority of patients we see in our specialized outpatient clinic, which has a focus on functional GI disorders, have previously consulted a doctor in primary care. The etiological and pathophysiological mechanisms in IBS are only partly understood, and there are no biological markers, which makes IBS a symptom-based diagnosis. Many patients express dissatisfaction with their earlier contacts with the healthcare system after having been told that "everything is okay," or "all tests and medical examinations are normal," and/or "no disease is found." These statements are not reassuring to most IBS patients who seek health care, as they still experience symptoms despite being told "everything is normal." As well, many patients feel insufficiently informed, because often they have not received any explanation regarding why they have their symptoms. Therefore, they choose to consult elsewhere in the healthcare system. In our experience, the majority of patients highly appreciate a thorough explanation regarding how it is possible to have such severe GI symptoms without anything being found wrong on routine examination or after diagnostic tests. Many IBS patients also express feelings that their symptoms have not been taken seriously by healthcare professionals. By tradition, many healthcare providers are primarily focused on finding the organic problem responsible for the symptoms and then treating it. If no such organic abnormality is found, this is unfortunately often interpreted by the patient as "everything is normal or OK," which is obviously not an optimal approach when managing patients with a chronic disorder such as IBS.

At our unit, besides pharmacological treatment options for reducing different IBS symptoms, we use different forms of nonpharmacologic management strategies for IBS. One example of this is a structured follow-up visit to the consulting physician after all investigations have been performed. Besides providing test results, the visit focuses on a thorough explanation regarding our current knowledge of symptom generation in IBS, which consists of a combination of altered gastrointestinal motility and visceral hypersensitivity together with psychosocial factors. The end result of all of these factors is the hallmark symptom of IBS (ie, abdominal pain [or discomfort]) in conjunction with altered bowel habits. This can usually be explained to patients in an easy and understandable way, using layman's terms. The aim is to illustrate for the patient, based on his or her level of education and understanding, the functional alterations in the gut, as well as the interactions between the gut and different parts of our nervous system, that lead to symptom generation and expression.

Another successful intervention is structured patient education in a group setting, containing both IBS information given by healthcare professionals and an opportunity to meet and discuss with other patients who have similar symptoms.[3] Food intake seems to be one important issue in the patients' perspective of the disorder that negatively affects the daily life of IBS patients. It has been demonstrated that symptom aggravation in relation to food intake contributes to substantial difficulties in social contacts and is associated with feelings of helplessness. This is a very common topic discussed by patients during the group meetings. Other important issues included in the education program are self-help strategies, the impact of psychosocial factors on gut symptoms, the association between gut symptoms and extra-intestinal symptoms, and the fact that IBS per se does not lead to any severe medical complications, despite its disturbing symptoms.

Evaluations of these management strategies reveal that the patients often feel better just by having a name for their disorder—several patients have not been informed that they have IBS, despite consulting several healthcare providers. Instead, they have received information about what they *do not* have (ie, cancer, inflammatory bowel disease, and other organic diseases). Moreover, as they understand that it is possible to have severe GI symptoms without having a serious disease, much of their worries about the possible seriousness of their symptoms disappear. Most of our patients state that they first want information about what they can do to improve their daily symptoms followed by treatment options and causes of their symptoms.[4] This has also been demonstrated by others. Another study reports that IBS patients gain more confidence from getting advice about lifestyle modifications than they do from drugs.

Summary

Healthcare seeking in IBS is affected by the severity of gastrointestinal and psychological symptoms, as well as by the presence and severity of extra-intestinal symptoms and social factors. To reduce health-care consumption in these individuals, an effective and mutual interaction between the patients and the health-care provider is crucial, including a thorough explanation, reassurance, and a cost-effective evaluation, in which the patient is actively involved in all key decisions.

References

1. Whitehead WE, Levy RL, Von Korff M, et al. The usual medical care for irritable bowel syndrome. *Aliment Pharmacol Ther.* 2004;20(11-12):1305-1315.
2. Ringström G, Abrahamsson H, Strid H, Simrén M. Why do subjects with irritable bowel syndrome seek health care for their symptoms? *Scand J Gastroenterol.* 2007;42(10):1194-1203.
3. Ringström G, Störsrud S, Posserud I, Lundqvist S, Westman B, Simrén M. Structured patient education is superior to written information in the management of patients with irritable bowel syndrome: a randomized controlled study. *Eur J Gastroenterol Hepatol.* 2010;22(4):420-428.
4. Ringström G, Agerforz P, Lindh A, Jerlstad P, Wallin J, Simrén M. What do patients with irritable bowel syndrome know about their disorder and how do they use their knowledge? *Gastroenterol Nurs.* 2009;32(4):284-292.

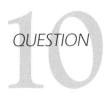

QUESTION

WHAT DISTINGUISHES A PATIENT WITH MILD IBS FROM A PATIENT WITH SEVERE IBS?

Filippo Cremonini, MD, MSc, PhD

Intrinsic to the definition of irritable bowel syndrome (IBS) is the fact that this chronic condition does not convey a grim prognosis. Conversely, an enormous amount of literature attests to the tremendous impact of IBS on patients' quality of life and also to society as a whole, with regard to the negative effects on work productivity and healthcare resource utilization. This chapter will address IBS severity, how it affects patients, and how physicians can effectively treat these patients.

The majority of referrals to a gastroenterology practice are for complaints compatible with a prospective IBS diagnosis. In general, both primary-care providers and specialists have increasingly become both comfortable and familiar with the need for a more conservative, minimalistic approach to IBS with regard to diagnostic testing. A number of studies have now shown that extensive testing in IBS patients is unlikely to either yield a new diagnosis or reassure the patient (see Chapters 6 and 7). However, in at least 19% of patients with underlying IBS,[1] healthcare providers are confronted with the clinical scenario of a patient with severe IBS symptoms, based on clinical symptoms, psychosocial factors, and overall burden to the patient. This may then force the clinician into a more elaborate, and time- and resource-consuming, diagnostic approach.

Studies of multicenter IBS registries have calculated disease-targeted utilities and measures of health-related quality of life and have found that severe IBS burden can parallel the burden from other, even life-threatening, chronic conditions, such as class III heart failure and rheumatoid arthritis.[2] Often, the distinction between mild, moderate, and severe IBS patients is blurred, and a systematic, proactive approach from the practicing clinician helps to identify potentially more problematic cases at the time of the initial office visit.

Some experienced gastroenterologists state they can recognize severe IBS, or at least potentially difficult-to-treat patients, at first glance, and most would be able to anecdotally describe a series of nonverbal clues or patient statements collected at the time of the initial office visit that would help classify these more difficult patients. While empiric approaches are part of the repertoire of each individual physician's art of practicing medicine, an effort should be made to rely on more objective, reproducible endpoints to facilitate appropriate patient triage and decision making.

How Should We Define IBS Severity?

Given the overall lack of biological markers for IBS in evidence-based practice and given the benign, yet difficult to predict, natural history, it is essential to focus on information that might point to a greater symptomatic burden over the patient's lifetime. Clinical trials have shifted from targeting the predominant bowel habit (ie, constipation or diarrhea) toward composite, global outcomes and patient-reported outcomes. Mounting evidence suggests that patient perception of disease severity is often not associated with more severe individual gastrointestinal symptoms.[3]

Prior to administering and interpreting formal instruments for the assessment of IBS severity, a few limitations must be borne in mind. First, results should be put in the context of a limited time window. As IBS symptoms often fluctuate over time, a reliable estimate of severity requires a prolonged observation. Unfortunately, most patients cannot accurately recall symptoms or events from weeks or months earlier, and thus significant recall bias can occur. Second, estimates of severity can vary widely between the patient and physician. A potential way to circumvent this shortcoming is to review and reconcile the results of a standardized questionnaire during the office interview. This questionnaire can be filled out by the patient before the office visit, which will also make the visit more efficient.

Two popular measuring tools for severity in IBS are the IBS Severity Scoring System (IBS-SSS) and the Functional Bowel Disease Severity Index (FBDSI; Table 10-1).[4,5] The IBS-SSS incorporates measures of pain, distension, bowel dysfunction, and quality of life/well-being. The FBDSI questionnaire combines pain ratings using a visual analog scale, in a formula obtained from a regression function. Similar to other numeric scales used by clinicians to assess other chronic medical conditions, such as diabetes and osteoarthritis, these scales have proven to have clinical responsiveness. That is, these scales vary according to significant clinical changes in patients' status. In addition, these scales have been shown to have both construct and convergent validity. Thus, they remain reliable across the wide spectrum of IBS patients, are consistent with prospective clinical trial experience, and reliably predict resource utilization, at least in the short term. A relevant aspect of the severity scales is that they shift the paradigm from the centrality of bowel habits to a combination of features that can be easily and specifically addressed during the patient encounter.

While approaches used in clinical trials cannot be automatically extrapolated to the office setting, the lesson learned is that patient perceptions of symptoms and other issues related to the diagnosis of IBS can directly conflict with objective data regarding the frequency and form of bowel habits and measurements used to accurately record abdominal pain. However, these perceptions constitute an important endpoint that cannot be ignored by the clinician if treatment is to be successful.

Several symptom- and health-related quality of life questionnaires have been validated and are routinely used in the research arena. We routinely administer a short, yet

Table 10-1

The Two Most Commonly Used Scales for Quantifying IBS Severity

Scale	Endpoints Included	Score Calculation	Categories	Validation	Potential Limitations
IBS-Severity Scoring System (IBS-SSS)	Pain, distension, bowel dysfunction, quality of life/global well-being over 10-day period	Score 0 to 100 per item, aggregate scores	75 to 175, mild 175 to 300, moderate >300, severe	Clinical trials Large prospective cohorts	Less reliable if symptoms fluctuate
Functional Bowel Disease Severity Index (FBDSI)	Patient rating of pain by VAS, number of physician visits in previous 6 months, disabling features combined in a formula	Composite of 0 to 100 for pain VAS, 1 or 0 for functional disorder diagnosis ×106, number of doctor visits ×11	<37, mild 37 to 110, moderate >110, severe	Clinical trials Large prospective cohorts	No inclusion of specific bowel symptoms More descriptive of longer time spans (6 months)

comprehensive general gastrointestinal symptom form with questions pertaining to psychological and somatization aspects, along with questions extrapolated from quality-of-life questionnaires, such as the 12-item short form (SF-12) prior to the encounter. Consistently incorporating key items of these questionnaires in the clinical interview might also work for the busy clinician. The involvement of patients in the direct documentation of their symptoms can increase self-awareness of the condition and, potentially, can provide some insight into what specific symptoms patients are seeking to improve.

It is worth emphasizing the increased attention that the symptom of pain has received in the development of novel treatments for IBS, as at least some of this focus should be incorporated into practice. This is highlighted by the fact that, in view of the failure of a number of experimental drugs in clinical trials, the US Food and Drug Administration (FDA) has recently moved toward recommending that pain be considered a central, strategic endpoint in IBS clinical trials. Pain appears to be a strong predictor of patient status and healthcare seeking and can be used to measure severity regardless of the predominant bowel habit.[6,7] Clinicians, however, frequently disagree as to whether pain is the prominent feature in the majority of patients.

The relative impact of pain is still an object of ongoing research, yet scales for measuring pain, often borrowed from other subspecialties, have been validated in IBS. Validated pain numeric scales have been linked, in a large, longitudinal cohort of IBS, with lesser quality of life, work productivity, and several individual bowel symptoms, but not with bowel frequency or stool form, which many clinicians still commonly use as the key IBS symptom.

In our practice, we tend to regard patients with predominant pain as more severe, and we tend to associate them with the need for more invasive tests, imaging, emergency room visits, use of narcotics, multiple return appointments, contacts with multiple colleagues, and repeated phone calls.

Psychological comorbidities are another major aspect that needs to be recognized as early as possible in the evaluation of a patient with severe IBS symptoms. The impact of depression, anxiety, abuse, and somatization on IBS symptoms has been extensively characterized. Surprisingly, published studies are not in complete agreement that these conditions lead to increased healthcare resources in IBS, although most of the research has been done in tertiary centers. Nonetheless, we strongly recommend the early recognition of psychological issues in IBS patients, with referral to the appropriate specialist for treatment of these comorbid conditions that exist in parallel with GI symptoms. We also recommend that a portion of the encounter be spent discussing extra-intestinal symptoms of IBS. While the association of IBS with fibromyalgia has been recognized for years and primary-care physicians are well aware of it, other, more subtle factors can predict a more burdensome course of IBS. Some of these symptoms, such as fatigue, low energy levels, sleep disturbance, sexual dysfunction, and overall concern about health, can be isolated and not part of a defined psychological diagnosis. These and other symptoms have been strongly associated with a more disruptive IBS course, thus once more reinforcing the need to go beyond the identification of bowel habits during the clinical assessment.

Does IBS Severity Reflect a Distinct Underlying Biological Basis?

Perturbations in motility and sensation, central modulation of afferent and efferent stimuli, along with psychosocial and biological (eg, previous gastroenteritis, microflora, diet) factors have all been recognized as components of a biopsychosocial model for the pathogenesis of IBS.[8] None of these factors has been independently identified as associated with a more severe presentation. It is plausible that the number of deranged mechanisms would be proportional to the severity of symptoms; however, no study has formally tackled this complicated issue in IBS.

Gender differences in IBS are often described, with the majority of patients referred to specialist care being female, as reflected by clinical trials participation. As discussed in Chapter 17, it is not uncommon for many women to report a worsening of their symptoms during menses. A recent meta-analysis of 22 studies concluded that gender differences in IBS do exist; however, the differences appeared to be modest.[9]

The search for genetic determinants of IBS continues. The association of IBS phenotypes with genetic polymorphisms for the serotonin transporter, cannabinoid, cholecystokinin, and beta-adrenergic receptors, G-proteins, and various interleukins has been tested. However, results are not unequivocal, partly owing to variability in tested populations, and there is no clear suggestion that individuals with IBS harboring any of these polymorphisms tend to present with greater severity or have a different natural history. The quest for candidate molecular markers continues, although it appears unlikely that a single factor, be it biological or not, would be responsible for more than a small amount of phenotypic variability in a large group of patients. Rather, the gain of deeper insight into IBS epigenetics, that is, the interaction between the environment and genetic predisposition, may further our understanding.[10]

Do Some Severe IBS Patients Deserve a More Aggressive Approach?

Finding the right balance between excessive testing and immediately discounting the severe symptoms as functional, chronic, and innocuous is probably the single most important clinical skill in the management of IBS. It is unclear the extent to which healthcare utilization is related to patients' expectations and to physicians' knowledge and attitudes. Many providers have attempted to design a roadmap toward more conservative testing; however, the decision largely remains at the discretion of the individual practitioner. The traditional approach of looking for "alarm symptoms" can discriminate IBS from organic lower gastrointestinal conditions, even if the reverse approach, that of using alarm symptoms to screen for organic conditions, has potential fallacies.[11] A proposed algorithm for the management of patients with severe IBS is presented in Figure 10-1.

Prior to formulating a therapeutic plan, it is essential to set realistic expectations and goals regarding the potential improvement of symptoms, recognizing that IBS is a chronic condition of poorly understood etiology for which no definitive therapeutic intervention has been identified.

Once the diagnosis is fully established, the issue remains whether patients with a more severe presentation deserve a more aggressive, nonstepwise approach. Similar to what is evolving practice in other fields of gastroenterology, including inflammatory bowel disease (IBD), a more aggressive (eg, "top-down") approach could be conceived for patients with severe IBS manifestations. This approach also needs to take into account that it is unlikely that such patients would present naïve of any of the innumerable empirical treatments available over the counter, from herbal laxatives to probiotics. In the average patient with mild symptoms, our approach has been more conservative. That is, we start treatment with nonprescription medications and remedies and gradually add agents with more potential systemic effects and a less favorable side effect profile.

Although multiple reasons have prevented conducting rigorous trials comparing combinations of drugs, in real life, single agents or unimodal approaches do not achieve satisfactory symptom control in severe IBS. One could thus envision, as an example, that in patients with severe constipation-predominant IBS, significant pain, coexisting anxiety, and somatization, treatment would start with a combination of laxatives along with a chloride channel activator or a Guanylate C-receptor agonist, the use of a tricyclic

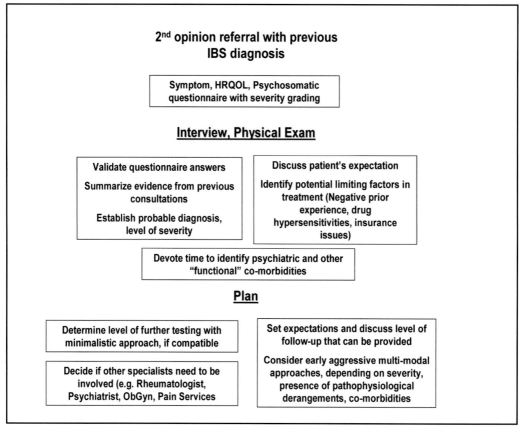

Figure 10-1. A proposed practice algorithm for the evaluation of an IBS patient with severe IBS symptoms.

antidepressant to control visceral pain, cognitive behavioral therapy to improve overall well-being, and the initiation of biofeedback for coexisting pelvic floor dysfunction. In academic and tertiary centers, enrollment in a clinical trial is a further option that is frequently offered, especially if multiple standard treatments fail.

The main caveat to such an approach is that, in IBD and rheumatoid arthritis, there is evidence that the newer biological agents favorably modify the natural history of the disease. This does not hold true for IBS, which is a nonlife-threatening condition, thus narrowing the benefit/risk ratio, especially with off-label use of medications. However, the careful choice of an aggressive, multimodal approach in selected, severe IBS patients could succeed in reducing the disease burden to the individual, his or her family, and to society.

References

1. Lembo A, Ameen VZ, Drossman DA. Irritable bowel syndrome: toward an understanding of severity. *Clin Gastroenterol Hepatol.* 2005;3:717-725.
2. Spiegel B, Harris L, Lucak S, et al. Developing valid and reliable health utilities in irritable bowel syndrome: results from the IBS PROOF Cohort. *Am J Gastroenterol.* 2009;104:1984-1991.

3. Hahn BA, Kirchdoerfer LJ, Fullerton S, et al. Patient-perceived severity of irritable bowel syndrome in relation to symptoms, health resource utilization and quality of life. *Aliment Pharmacol Ther.* 1997;11:553-559.

4. Drossman DA, Li Z, Toner BB, et al. Functional bowel disorders. A multicenter comparison of health status and development of illness severity index. *Dig Dis Sci.* 1995;40:986-995.

5. Francis CY, Morris J, Whorwell PJ. The irritable bowel severity scoring system: a simple method of monitoring irritable bowel syndrome and its progress. *Aliment Pharmacol Ther.* 1997;11:395-402.

6. Sandler RS, Drossman DA, Nathan HP, et al. Symptom complaints and health care seeking behavior in subjects with bowel dysfunction. *Gastroenterology.* 1984;87:314-318.

7. Whitehead WE, Crowell MD, Bosmajian L, et al. Existence of irritable bowel syndrome supported by factor analysis of symptoms in two community samples. *Gastroenterology.* 1990;98:336-340.

8. Cremonini F, Talley NJ. Treatments targeting putative mechanisms in irritable bowel syndrome. *Nat Clin Pract Gastroenterol Hepatol.* 2005;2:82-88.

9. Adeyemo MA, Spiegel BM, Chang L. Meta-analysis: do irritable bowel syndrome symptoms vary between men and women? *Aliment Pharmacol Ther.* 2010;32(6):738-755.

10. Saito YA, Mitra N, Mayer EA. Genetic approaches to functional gastrointestinal disorders. *Gastroenterology.* 2010;138:1276-1285.

11. Hammer J, Eslick GD, Howell SC, et al. Diagnostic yield of alarm features in irritable bowel syndrome and functional dyspepsia. *Gut.* 2004;53:666-672.

WHY IS IBS IMPORTANT TO TREAT?

Brennan M. R. Spiegel, MD, MSHS

Irritable bowel syndrome (IBS) is common, significantly impacts quality of life, limits work productivity, and is even associated with suicidality.[1-4] For all these reasons, it is vital to understand how to identify and effectively treat this condition. To better appreciate the importance of effective treatments for IBS, which is covered in more detail elsewhere in this book, it is first useful to understand the latest information about IBS burden of illness. This chapter reviews the relevant data about the epidemiology and quality-of-life impact of IBS and provides additional information about practical ways to address the burden of this disease in the clinic.

Irritable bowel syndrome can affect patients physically, psychologically, socially, and economically. Knowledge about this burden of illness serves several purposes. For patients, it emphasizes that many others have IBS and that people suffering from the disorder should not feel alone with their diagnosis or disease-related experiences. For healthcare providers, it highlights the fact that IBS makes up a significant part of their practices and emphasizes the need to understand the disease more fully in order to appropriately mange their patients. Moreover, it allows providers to improve their understanding of the impact of IBS on their patients' well-being and then act on this knowledge by selecting treatments tailored to each patient's unique symptoms and health-related quality-of-life (HRQOL) decrement. For research funding and drug-approval authorities like the Food and Drug Administration, it points out that IBS is more than a mere nuisance condition and is instead a syndrome with a prevalence and illness impact that matches other common diagnoses like diabetes, hypertension, or kidney disease.[1,2] Lastly, for employers and healthcare insurers, it reveals the overwhelming direct and indirect expenditures related to IBS and provides a business rationale to ensure that IBS is treated effectively.[1-7]

Several studies have compared HRQOL in IBS patients with HRQOL in healthy controls or controls with non-IBS medical disorders.[6,7] Patients with IBS have the same physical HRQOL as patients with diabetes and a lower physical HRQOL compared with patients who have depression or gastroesophageal reflux disease.[6,7] Perhaps more surprisingly, mental HRQOL scores were lower in patients with IBS than in those with chronic renal failure—an organic condition marked by considerable physical and mental disability. This HRQOL decrement can, in some cases, be so severe as to raise the risk of suicidal behavior. The relationship between IBS and suicidality is independent of comorbid psychiatric diseases such as depression.[3] Many of these studies were performed in tertiary-care referral populations, and the HRQOL decrement and suicidality risk documented in these cohorts may not be applicable to community-based populations. Nonetheless, IBS unquestionably has a negative impact on HRQOL, and failing to recognize this impact could undermine the physician-patient relationship and lead to dissatisfaction with care. Because HRQOL decrements are common in IBS patients, clinicians should perform routine screening for diminished HRQOL in their IBS patients. Treatment should be initiated when the symptoms of IBS are found to reduce functional status and diminish overall HRQOL. Furthermore, clinicians should remain wary of potential suicidal behavior in patients with severe IBS symptoms and should initiate timely interventions if suicide forerunners are identified.

A practical limitation of determining HRQOL in the busy outpatient setting is that its accurate measurement requires a thorough and often time-consuming evaluation of biologic, psychologic, and social health domains. To help providers gain better insight into their patients' HRQOL, a concise list of factors known to predict HRQOL in IBS might be helpful, which providers could then use to question patients routinely. Indeed, several studies have identified predictors of HRQOL in IBS, the most consistent of which is the intensity of abdominal pain. Data from several studies indicate that in patients with IBS, HRQOL decreases in parallel with increasing pain intensity. It is therefore important not only to identify the presence of pain in IBS patients, but also to gauge its intensity using a standard 0-10 numeric rating scale. Additional data indicate that *physical* HRQOL in IBS is associated with the duration of symptom flares ($\geq$ 24 hours versus < 24 hours) and *mental* HRQOL is associated with abnormalities in sexuality, mood, and anxiety. Perhaps more importantly, both domains share a common association with symptoms of chronic stress and vital exhaustion, including tiring easily, feeling low in energy, and experiencing sleep difficulties. Patients acknowledge that these symptoms prompt avoidance of socially vulnerable situations (eg, being away from restrooms) and activities (eg, eating out for dinner). In contrast, HRQOL is not strongly determined by the presence of specific gastrointestinal symptoms (eg, diarrhea, constipation, bloating, dyspepsia), degree of previous gastrointestinal evaluation (eg, previous flexible sigmoidoscopy or colonoscopy), or common demographic characteristics (eg, gender, age, marital status).

The above findings suggest that, rather than focusing on physiological epiphenomena to gauge HRQOL (eg, stool frequency, stool characteristics, subtype of IBS), it may be more efficient to assess HRQOL by gauging global symptom severity, addressing symptom-related fears and concerns, and identifying and eliminating factors contributing to vital exhaustion in IBS. This process may occur through teaching coping mechanisms and relaxation skills, developing a greater sense of self-efficacy by encouraging control over IBS symptoms, promoting appropriate lifestyle modifications (ie, diet, exercise, quitting smoking), and allowing patients to recognize their own limitations.[8-10] When provided in concert with standard medical therapies, these approaches yield improved overall HRQOL. In short, treating bowel symptoms alone in IBS is necessary, but may not be sufficient, to impact overall HRQOL. In addition to treating symptoms, providers should attempt to positively modify the cognitive interpretation of IBS symptoms. Stated another way, healthcare providers need to acknowledge and address the emotional context in which IBS symptoms occur.

It is also important to treat IBS because patients with ongoing symptoms consume a disproportionate amount of resources. Burden of illness studies estimate that there are 3.6 million physician visits in the United States annually for IBS and that IBS care consumes more than $20 billion in both direct and indirect expenditures. Moreover, patients with IBS consume 50% more healthcare resources than matched controls without IBS. These data suggest that the economic burden of IBS stems not only from the high prevalence of the disease, but also from the disproportionate use of resources it causes.[11-13]

In addition to direct costs of care, IBS patients engender significant indirect costs of care as a consequence of both missing work and suffering impaired work performance while on the job. Employees with IBS are absent 3% to 5% of the workweek and report impaired productivity 26% to 31% of the week. These rates exceed those of non-IBS control employees by 20%, and this is equivalent to 14 hours of lost productivity per 40-hour workweek. Compared with IBS patients who exhibit normal work productivity, patients with impaired productivity have more extraintestinal comorbidities (eg, chronic fatigue syndrome, fibromyalgia, interstitial cystitis) and more disease-specific fears and concerns.[14-17] In contrast, the specific profile of individual bowel symptoms does not undermine work productivity, suggesting that enhancing work productivity in patients with IBS may require treatments that improve both GI and non-GI symptom intensity, while also modifying the cognitive and behavioral responses to bowel symptoms and the contexts in which they occur. In other words, it may be inadequate to treat bowel symptoms alone without simultaneously addressing the emotional context in which the symptoms occur.

References

1. El-Serag HB, Olden K, Bjorkaman D. Health-related quality of life among persons with irritable bowel syndrome: a systematic review. *Aliment Pharmacol Ther.* 2002;16:1171-1185.
2. American College of Gastroenterology Functional Gastrointestinal Disorders Task Force. Evidence-based position statement on the management of irritable bowel syndrome in North America. *Am J Gastroenterol.* 2002;97:S1-S2.
3. Spiegel BMR, Schoenfeld P, Naliboff B. Prevalence of suicidal behavior in patients with chronic abdominal pain and irritable bowel syndrome: a systematic review. *Aliment Pharmacol Ther.* 2007;26:183-193.
4. Hahn B, Kirchdoerfer L, Fullerton S, Mayer E. Patient-perceived severity of irritable bowel syndrome in relation to symptoms, health resource utilization, and quality of life. *Aliment Pharmacol Ther.* 1997;11:553-559.
5. Naliboff BD, Balice G, Mayer EA. Psychosocial moderators of quality of life in irritable bowel syndrome. *Eur J Surg Suppl.* 1998;583:57-59.
6. Creed F, Ratcliffe J, Fernandez L, et al. Health-related quality of life and health care costs in severe, refractory irritable bowel syndrome. *Ann Intern Med.* 2001;134:860-868.
7. Spiegel BM, Gralnek IM, Bolus R, et al. Clinical determinants of health-related quality of life in patients with irritable bowel syndrome. *Arch Intern Med.* 2004;164:1773-1780.
8. van der Veek PP, van Rood YR, Masclee AA. Clinical trial: short- and long-term benefit of relaxation training for irritable bowel syndrome. *Aliment Pharmacol Ther.* 2007;26:943-952.
9. Shaw G, Srivastava ED, Sadlier M, Swann P, James JY, Rhodes J. Stress management for irritable bowel syndrome: a controlled trial. *Digestion.* 1991;50:36-42.
10. Spiegel BMR, Naliboff B, Mayer E, Bolus R, Gralnek I, Shekelle P. The effectiveness of a model physician-patient relationship versus usual care in irritable bowel syndrome: a randomized controlled trial. *Gastroenterology.* 2006;130:A773.
11. American Gastroenterological Association Publication. The burden of gastrointestinal diseases. Bethesda, MD: American Gastroenterological Association Press; 2001.
12. Talley NJ, Gabriel SE, Harmsen WS, Zinsmeister AR, Evans RW. Medical costs in community subjects with irritable bowel syndrome. *Gastroenterology.* 1995;109:1736-1741.
13. Longstreth GF, Wilson A, Knight K, et al. Irritable bowel syndrome, health care use, and costs: a U.S. managed care perspective. *Am J Gastroenterol.* 2003;98:600-607.

14. Whitehead WE, Palsson O, Jones KR. Systematic review of the comorbidity of irritable bowel syndrome with other disorders: what are the causes and implications? *Gastroenterology.* 2002;122:1140-1156.

15. Pare P, Gray J, Lam S, et al. Health-related quality of life, work productivity, and health care resource utilization of subjects with irritable bowel syndrome: baseline results from LOGIC (Longitudinal Outcomes Study of Gastrointestinal Symptoms in Canada), a naturalistic study. *Clin Ther.* 2006;28:1726-1735.

16. Dean BB, Aquilar D, Barghout V, et al. Impairment in work productivity and health-related quality of life in patients with IBS. *Am J Managed Care.* 2005;11:S17-S26.

17. Spiegel BMR, Harris L, Lucak S, et al. Predictors of work productivity in irritable bowel syndrome (IBS): results from the PROOF Cohort. *Gastroenterology.* 2008;134:AB157.

SECTION III

THE PATHOPHYSIOLOGY OF IBS

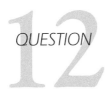

WHAT IS THE PATHOPHYSIOLOGY OF IBS?

Lisa Shim, MB BS, FRACP and John E. Kellow, MD, FRACP

Although irritable bowel syndrome (IBS) is one of the most common gastrointestinal disorders, its actual cause remains unknown. Over the past decades, however, new areas of research have improved our understanding of IBS considerably and have provided increasing evidence that its pathophysiology is complex and multifactorial. Today, IBS is no longer considered merely a psychosomatic condition but is best understood from a biopsychosocial perspective characterized by prominent dysregulation of the brain-gut axis.

Dysregulation of the Brain-Gut Axis

The central nervous system communicates with the enteric nervous system of the gut via sympathetic and parasympathetic pathways in a bidirectional circuit. Using sophisticated techniques such as functional magnetic resonance imaging (fMRI) and positron emission tomography (PET), some IBS patients appear to have abnormal cortical responses to gut stimulation.[1] On the other hand, mood changes such as anxiety and depression have been found to influence the autonomic nervous system and gut motility and sensation.[2] Thus, dysregulation within the neural circuitry of the brain-gut axis is now regarded as an important overarching concept underlying the pathophysiology of IBS symptoms. Established pathophysiological factors related to this dysregulation are altered gastrointestinal motility, abnormal gas handling, visceral hypersensitivity, and psychosocial dysfunction, with emerging evidence for a role for genetic factors, alterations in gut neurotransmitters, infections, microscopic gut inflammation and immune activation, and altered gut microflora (Figure 12-1).

Altered Gut Motility

A range of motor abnormalities have been described in the small bowel and colon of patients with IBS.[3] In particular, several studies have shown an increased frequency of

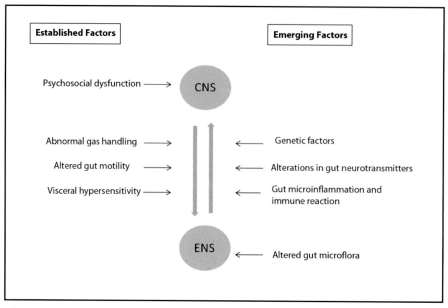

Figure 12-1. Putative pathophysiological factors associated with brain-gut dysregulation in IBS.

high-amplitude propagating contractions in the colon in IBS patients, some of which can be associated with abdominal cramping pain. An exaggerated postprandial myoelectrical and motor response in these patients has also been demonstrated. Altered gut transit may be important in determining bowel habits. Patients with diarrhea-predominant IBS have been found to have rapid transit through the small bowel and colon, whereas those with constipation-predominant IBS appear to have slower transit. Overall, these studies support a link between gastrointestinal motor dysfunction and the symptoms of IBS.

Abnormal Gas Handling

Bloating and abdominal distension are common complaints of IBS patients. These symptoms have not been reliably shown to be related to an increased total volume of gas within the gastrointestinal tract compared to healthy subjects. There is evidence, however, to suggest that IBS patients have impaired gut transit and do not expel gas as efficiently as healthy subjects (see Chapter 14). Furthermore, impaired coordination of the abdominal wall and diaphragmatic muscles as well as abnormal gastrointestinal reflex activity have been found to be present in IBS patients with bloating and distension.

Visceral Hypersensitivity

A number of balloon distension studies in the gut have shown that a high proportion of IBS patients experience pain and discomfort at a lower distending volume and pressure compared to healthy subjects.[3] This visceral hypersensitivity, demonstrable by assessing rectal sensitivity, is one of the most reproducible physiologic markers for IBS. Visceral hypersensitivity can be exacerbated in association with certain stimuli, such as food intake and stress, consistent with IBS patients' reports of worsening of symptoms at these times. The precise mechanism underlying visceral hypersensitivity remains unknown. However, both central and peripheral factors are likely to be contributory.

Psychosocial Factors

It is known that IBS patients tend to have underlying comorbid psychological conditions that are independent of healthcare seeking behaviors.[4] Up to 50% of IBS patients may suffer from psychiatric dysfunction with the most common associations being depression, anxiety, panic disorder, and somatization. Such psychologic comorbidities may be a risk factor for developing IBS and may determine the severity of IBS symptoms. A history of childhood sexual or physical abuse has also been linked to IBS and appears to be associated with increased symptom reporting. Therefore, identification of these factors and initiation of appropriate counseling or psychotherapy is important in the overall management of IBS patients.

Genetic Factors

Patients with IBS often report that their family members also suffer from the same condition. A recent population-based study showed that relatives of IBS subjects were threefold more likely to have IBS than controls. Twin studies have suggested that up to 20% of IBS results from genetic contribution. However, no one specific gene has yet been identified, and the influence of environmental factors remains a confounding issue. Overall, these studies have highlighted that genetic as well as environmental contributions may be important in IBS.

Neuropeptides and Hormones

Several chemical neurotransmitters have been shown to be involved in the alteration of sensory and motor dysfunction in the gut of IBS patients. These include neuropeptide Y, vasoactive intestinal peptide, cholecystokinin, and motilin; the clinical significance of alterations in these gut peptides has not been established. The main research focus has been on serotonin (5-HT), which is one of the key signaling molecules within the gastrointestinal tract.[4] Both local and blood levels of serotonin have been shown to be increased in diarrhea-predominant IBS patients, whereas reduced levels are seen in those with constipation-predominant IBS. As a result, several therapies that target 5-HT receptors have been developed to treat IBS.

Gut Inflammation and Microflora

Up to 25% of patients report symptoms of IBS after an enteric infection. Studies have demonstrated an increased number of T-lymphocytes, mast cells, and enteroendocrine cells in the colonic mucosa of IBS patients, especially those with postinfective IBS. These inflammatory cells are capable of influencing motor and sensory responses in the gut via mediators such as interleukins and nitric oxide. However, the precise mechanism by which microscopic gut inflammation could result in symptom generation remains unclear.

Several studies have reported alterations in indigenous gut microflora as a potential etiology in IBS by inducing gut mucosal irritation and inflammation.[4] Decreased levels of *Coliforms, Lactobacilli,* and *Bifidobacteria* have been demonstrated in IBS patients. These types of studies have led to the possible therapeutic role of probiotics, which have been shown in some studies to improve symptoms of bloating and flatulence in IBS patients. There are also studies, using lactulose hydrogen breath testing, that suggest an increase in small bowel bacterial overgrowth in IBS patients. Subsequent studies have demonstrated an improvement of symptoms with antibiotics in these patients. However, the results are inconsistent, and the findings remain controversial. Overall, the role of gut inflammation and microflora in IBS needs to be further explored.

What Does This Mean to the Patient?

It is important to reassure the patient that IBS is not merely a psychological disorder, but a complex condition with disrupted communication between the brain and gut. This "disruption" may be due to a number of factors, such as genetics, emotional stress, abnormal motility and sensation of the bowel, chemical imbalances in the gut, and infections. Altogether, these factors may contribute to symptoms of abdominal pain and abnormal bowel function that are typical of IBS patients. The integration of these factors into routine consultations forms an important part of the overall management of IBS patients. A better understanding of this chronic condition will help reduce feelings of frustration and isolation commonly associated with the lack of knowledge and support among IBS sufferers.

Summary

IBS is a complex disorder with multiple etiologies. Several pathophysiological factors clearly play an important role in generating symptomatology in IBS. More importantly, it is the interactions between these factors that are responsible for the altered motor and sensory responses that most directly relate to the symptoms of abdominal pain and altered bowel habit. Continuing elucidation of these interactions will help develop appropriate management strategies for this very common yet distressing condition.

References

1. Van Oudenhove L, Aziz Q. Recent insights on central processing and psychological processes in functional gastrointestinal disorders. *Dig Liver Dis.* 2009;41:781 787.
2. Camilleri M, Mckinzie S, Busciglio I, et al. Prospective study of motor, sensory, psychologic, and autonomic functions in patients with irritable bowel syndrome. *Clin Gastroenterol Hepatol.* 2008;6:772-781.
3. Gunnarsson J, Simren M. Peripheral factors in the pathophysiology of irritable bowel syndrome. *Dig Liver Dis.* 2009;41:788-793.
4. Barbara G, De Giorgio R, Stanghellini V, Cremon C, Salvioli B, Corinaldesi R. New pathophysiological mechanisms in irritable bowel syndrome. *Aliment Pharmacol Ther.* 2004;20:1-9.

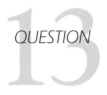
ARE THERE RISK FACTORS FOR DEVELOPING IBS?

Peter Paine, MD, PhD, MRCP and Lesley A. Houghton, PhD, FSB, FACG, AGAF

What might be a risk factor for IBS is highly inter-related to its possible cause. To date, however, a precise cause has remained elusive, although multiple possible interactions have been identified. It is, therefore, not surprising that there are a number of potential risk factors for the development of IBS.

Identification of these possible risk factors has come primarily from epidemiology studies, from twin/family studies, from studying postinfectious IBS (PI-IBS), and from information gleaned from preclinical human and animal models of IBS.

Given the etiological heterogeneity of IBS, efforts to characterize a more defined phenotype have largely focused on postinfectious IBS (PI-IBS).[1] Although it must be remembered that PI-IBS only comprises a small subset of IBS (between 6% and 17% of all IBS in one series), a number of risk factors for the development of persistent symptoms have nonetheless emerged.

For example, the risk for developing PI-IBS appears to be greater in "Westernized" nations. Whether this reflects differential exposure to infections in earlier life or greater antibiotic use or some other environmental factor, such as diet, is unclear. It does not appear to be related to ethnicity.

Microbiological factors relating to the type of infective organism, the dose, its virulence, and the part of the bowel affected appear to play a role in the risk for persistence and type of symptoms in PI-IBS. The greater the severity of the infection, the greater appears to be the chance of developing PI-IBS, which may be reflected by the presence of persistent subclinical inflammation.

The constituents of the host microbiome also appear to influence the risk of developing PI-IBS, with studies showing evidence for "dysbiosis" in these patients (an altered balance of bowel flora away from lactobacilli and bifidobacteria in particular). However, the degree to which this is cause or effect and the influence that diet and antibiotics may have remain unclear.

The host's immune response also appears to affect the PI-IBS risk, and there is evidence for alterations in both the mucosal inflammatory and systemic cytokine responses in IBS patients. The debate is somewhat polarized as to the relevance of these modest inflammatory changes with some authorities considering IBS and IBD as extremes of a spectrum, while others consider the findings to be epiphenomenon.

Being female is a clear risk factor for developing IBS. This remains the case even after adjusting for differences between the sexes in seeking out a consultation. The reason for this is unclear but it is known that sex hormones can alter pain perception.

Psychological factors emerge consistently as strong risk factors for IBS. These include current psychological state, which is particularly influenced by recent adverse life stress events, and comorbid psychiatric disorders, especially anxiety and depression. The presence of other coexistent functional gastrointestinal and somatoform syndromes also represents a risk factor for developing subsequent IBS. Psychological traits, which are enduring stable personality traits, in particular anxiety and neuroticism, further modulate the risks of developing PI-IBS.

Adverse early life events are also thought to be risk factors for developing IBS later in life. The experience of childhood abuse, sexual and otherwise, is a well-documented predisposition for IBS, as well as severe childhood illness. Animal models demonstrate that severe stressors in early life can produce lifelong alterations in patterns of psychoneuroimmune and endocrine reactivity, which may mediate this vulnerability.[2]

Family studies have demonstrated increased familial IBS even when controlling for recent or early life infective/adverse events. However, twin studies have suggested that only a finite and probably minor proportion of this familial risk appears attributable to genetics, with the assumption that the larger proportion relates to learned behavior from other family members or other environmental factors.[3]

It is clear, therefore, that there are multiple possible risk factors for IBS in a number of different domains (eg, gender, immune, psychosocial, etc), none of which are mutually exclusive and which may interact in complex ways (Table 13-1). Interactions between psychological, immune, and genetic risk factors, for example, may be mediated through differences in central or autonomic neurohumoral processes. However, it seems likely that there needs to be more than one risk factor "hit" or "insult" before chronic healthcare seeking IBS symptoms begin to emerge. The biopsychosocial model is again a useful framework in this regard when considering the complexity, multiplicity, and interactions of risk factors in any individual.

Practically, in the clinic, some risk factors are more sensitive and difficult to explore with patients, particularly at the psychosocial end of the spectrum. It is also questionable how legitimate it is to do so unless a significant psychotherapeutic infrastructure is available, because some of these are difficult to modify with well-established symptoms far removed from precipitating events. The PI-IBS model, however, suggests it may be possible to risk stratify patients at the time of an infection or planned bowel injury (such as surgery). This could lead to more intensive intervention for those with the greatest cluster of risks with, for example, psychological therapies, probiotics, or immunomodulating agents. This hypothesis, however, remains to be tested before such clinical intervention could be recommended.

Table 13-1

Putative Risk Factors for the Development of IBS

- Western nations
- GI infection severity
- Altered bowel microflora
- Mucosal inflammatory activity
- Female gender
- Psychological state (stress, anxiety, depression)
- Psychological trait (neuroticism)
- Adverse early life events
- Family sick role behavior

References

1. Spiller R, Garsed K. Postinfectious irritable bowel syndrome. *Gastroenterology.* 2009;136(6):1979-1988.
2. Chitkara DK, van Tilburg MA, Blois-Martin N, Whitehead WE. Early life risk factors that contribute to irritable bowel syndrome in adults: a systematic review. *Am J Gastroenterol.* 2008;103(3):765-774; quiz 775.
3. Levy RL, Jones KR, Whitehead WE, Feld SI, Talley NJ, Corey LA. Irritable bowel syndrome in twins: heredity and social learning both contribute to etiology. *Gastroenterology.* 2001;121(4):799-804.

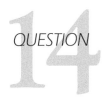
WHY IS BLOATING SUCH A PROBLEM IN PATIENTS WITH IBS?

Juan R. Malagelada, MD

Bloating is very common and, like other symptoms associated with irritable bowel syndrome (IBS), occurs in the general population, especially women, at relatively low levels of intensity or frequency that do not motivate medical consultation. Thus, the bloaters that we see in clinic tend to belong to one of two general categories: first, patients with rather severe bloating (or perceived by patients as severe), and, second, patients with IBS who describe bloating to the attending physician but who, in fact, are primarily motivated to consult because of the typical IBS symptoms of pain and altered bowel habit, rather than by bloating.[1]

Nevertheless, it is sometimes difficult in clinical practice to separate abdominal pain and bloating, as patients may refer to their bloating sensation as extremely uncomfortable, or even painful. In general, if patients describe bloating, even painful bloating, without the altered habit component that defines IBS, we tend to categorize them as functional bloating. Otherwise, we categorize them as bloating associated with IBS.

To complicate matters further, it is not uncommon for severe constipation to be associated with bloating. Fortunately, patients are usually able to distinguish the bloating that may develop during prolonged periods of fecal retention that improves with eventual defecation and the bloating that may be associated with constipation but that does not improve (or may even worsen) after defecation.

Patients are also generally able to characterize bloating associated with "gas retention" as it occurs, for instance, in situations (eg, work, social) that force individuals to restrain passing flatus for long periods of time. Conversely, they may describe bloating in association with increased flatulence. In this case, patients intuitively reject the notion that their bloating sensation may derive from excess gas retention.

Ultimately, clinicians must recognize that many combinations of symptoms may occur in a given patient with functional features and that the established definitions for IBS, functional bloating, and other categories contemplated in Rome III consensus are conventions based on group analysis. In day-to-day practice, there are many patients in the unclassifiable, mixed, or multiple syndrome categories.

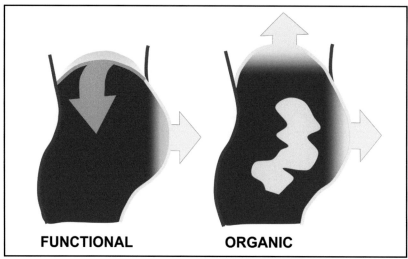

FUNCTIONAL   **ORGANIC**

Figure 14-1. Contrasting mechanisms of bloating in functional patients and intestinal dysmotility (organic).

When managing a patient with bloating, it is very important to keep in mind the two main mechanisms of bloating: abdominal reshaping and luminal retention of physical elements (gas, liquid, solid).

Abdominal reshaping is probably the commonest form of bloating. It appears to be produced by abnormal viscero-somatic reflex control of diaphragmatic and abdominal muscle activity. The psychological component may be crucial, as abdominal muscle tone is, at least partially, under voluntary control. Based on studies recently carried out in our laboratory, functional bloaters (with or without associated IBS) may indeed accumulate slightly higher amounts of gas in their bowels.[2,3] The amount of gas spontaneously retained by bloaters is often too small to create a perceptible difference in abdominal girth, but is sufficient to trigger an abnormal muscular response consisting of diaphragmatic descent and anterior oblique muscle relaxation (Figure 14-1). As a result, intra-abdominal volume may increase little or nothing, but the anterior abdomen becomes visibly protruded.[4] Increased visceral conscious perception is an important additional factor, because most bloated patients describe "feeling" not just "being" distended. Heightened perception of luminal distension of the small or large intestine is indeed a relevant feature of IBS, as verified by many studies.[5]

Another form of bloating, which is far less common, is that associated with significant gut neuromuscular dysfunction (neuropathy or myopathy) that causes massive gas retention in the bowel. These patients become distended, but their tolerance to retain gas is similar or even greater than normal individuals. Thus, sometimes, their abdominal distention is more obvious to the examiner than the discomfort they acknowledge. Aerophagics, that is individuals who swallow large quantities of air, may also voluntarily restrain anal evacuation and may end up with bowels massively filled up with gas, marked abdominal distention, and sometimes complaining of little or no abdominal discomfort.

Even though we have advanced considerably in our understanding of the pathophysiology of bloating in recent years, there are a number of features that may be associated with functional bloating, although the underlying mechanism remains uncertain. First, why do functional bloaters tend to feel more bloated late in the day than when they wake up in the morning? Also, why is bloating (also IBS) much more common in women than in men? What are the mechanisms by which affective disturbances influence functional symptoms like bloating?[6] Further research is required to elucidate these and other incompletely understood aspects of the bloating clinical picture.

From a patient perspective, the clinical relevance of bloating is compounded by social aspects. Besides the discomfort component, bloating entails image problems. Not uncommonly, patients acknowledge being fearful of the negative impression their distended abdomens may cause on other people; they may also acknowledge difficulties in wearing certain clothes, etc. The media, particularly commercial TV, tend to emphasize bloating as a lifestyle problem via advertisements of food and probiotics reputed to "cure" bloating.

Do we need to investigate bloating? The answer is not simple. It depends on its magnitude, duration, and impact on daily life activities of the consulting patient. Reassurance and minimal lifestyle counseling sometimes suffice, but severe bloating may need investigation for two main reasons. First, the patient may have an underlying gut neuromuscular disturbance that causes bloating via bowel distention with gas or fluid. Second, the patient may suffer from viscero-somatic dyssynergia that may be treatable by clear explanation of the symptom mechanism and biofeedback. Unfortunately, although the technology to elucidate these pathophysiological mechanisms in affected individuals does exist,[3,4,7] it is still only available for diagnostic testing in highly specialized centers with a research interest in gut motility disorders and their clinical evaluation.

References

1. Azpiroz F, Malagelada J-R. Abdominal bloating. *Gastroenterology.* 2005;129:1060-1078.
2. Salvioli B, Serra J, Azpiroz F, et al. Origin of gas retention and symptoms in patients with bloating. *Gastroenterology.* 2005;128:574-579.
3. Serra J, Villoria A, Azpiroz F, et al. Impaired intestinal gas propulsion in manometrically proven dysmotility and in irritable bowel syndrome. *Neurogastroenterol Mot.* 2010;22:401-406.
4. Accarino A, Perez F, Azpiroz F, Quiroga S, Malagelada JR. Abdominal distension results from caudo-ventral redistribution of contents. *Gastroenterology.* 2009;136:1544-1551.
5. Accarino A, Azpiroz F, Malagelada J-R. Modification of small bowel mechanosensitivity by intestinal fat. *Gut.* 2001;48:690-695.
6. Van Oudenhove L. The link between affective and functional gastrointestinal disorders: are we solving the psychobiological puzzle? *Neurogastroenterol Motil.* 2008;20:1265-1267.
7. Malagelada C, De Iorio F, Azpiroz F, et al. New insight into intestinal motor function via non-invasive endoluminal image analysis. *Gastroenterology.* 2008;135:1155-1162.

WHAT IS THE ROLE OF STRESS IN IBS?

Yvette Taché, PhD, and Agata Mulak, MD, PhD

The term *stress* was originally coined by Hans Selye in the early part of the past century to define the concept of "specific biological response of the organism to any demand." Over the years, ambiguity has surfaced from this definition in the scientific literature, and the term *stress* has been misused by the lay public and associated with emotional arousal or nervous tension. Our current understanding of stress involves the distinction between *stressors* and the *stress response*. Stressors are the internal or external stimuli/events threatening homeostasis or perceived as such. The *stress response* triggered by stressors is characterized by a complex repertoire of behavioral and physiological neuronal, endocrine, autonomic, and immune changes occurring in the brain and peripheral organs. Therefore, any kind of internal or external stimuli that results in physical, chemical, emotional, or psychological strain engages an organism's stressor-related adaptive homeostatic mechanisms. These mechanisms encompass changes in neuronal activity in interconnected brain regions, namely the hypothalamus, amygdala, hippocampus, and locus coeruleus, which receive input from higher cortical structures but also from visceral and somatic afferents. The stressor-activated central neural network causes behavioral manifestations. It also drives the autonomic nervous system (ANS) and neuroendocrine hypothalamic-pituitary-adrenal (HPA) axis efferent arms of the stress response, which impact the immune system and visceral organs. This stress response is adaptive in nature, however. Depending upon early life events, genetic or epigenetic background, and the magnitude and duration of the stressors, basal activity and/or responsiveness of the stress system may be altered (excessive, prolonged, or inadequate), leading to deleterious structural or functional changes, which can predispose an individual to develop or exacerbate a stress-sensitive disorder, such as irritable bowel syndrome (IBS).[1,2]

A great majority of IBS patients who are asked about the role of stress in the manifestation of their symptoms (abdominal pain, altered bowel habits) will respond affirmatively. Patients with IBS, when compared to healthy subjects, seem to be more affected by stress, at both the psychological and physiological levels. This may result from an increased exposure to stressors and/or altered responsiveness to stress. In fact, a history of early adverse life events in the form of physical, sexual, or emotional abuse, neglect, or early parental loss has been shown to be a major predisposing factor for the development of functional gastrointestinal disorders (eg, IBS) later in life. Childhood trauma, especially in genetically predisposed individuals, is thought to induce persistent changes in the central stress response systems, including the HPA axis. In addition, it may cause epigenetic programming of glucocorticoid receptor expression that affects behavioral adaptation and susceptibility to stress-related disorders. Furthermore, early life adversity is also associated with a poorer outcome and higher levels of distress in adult patients with IBS. In keeping with these clinical observations, animal models of maternal separation display HPA axis hyper-responsiveness, which predisposes adult rats to develop stress-related visceral hypersensitivity, increased colonic motility, and anxiety-like behavior. In adult IBS patients, exposure to acute stress episodes may additionally affect the onset, severity, and/or persistence of intestinal symptoms. Furthermore, chronic life stress is another powerful predictor of subsequent symptom intensity. Epidemiological data confirm a higher prevalence of IBS in patients with post-traumatic stress disorders (eg, in war veterans). While some severe stressful events are correlated with permanent alterations of stress responsiveness, other stressors (even daily hassles) may play a role as triggers or perpetuation factors, especially in predisposed individuals. It is also recognized that IBS symptoms, and the social/work constraints they often impose on patients, can cause additional emotional distress, creating a stress-symptoms-stress vicious circle.[2]

Female predominance in IBS patients (women outnumber men by approximately 2:1) is consistent with the observation that women are more susceptible to stress-related disorders. A number of clinical and experimental studies have documented gender differences in the stress response and stress-induced pain modulation. It has been confirmed that sex hormones, in particular estrogens, can strongly affect the HPA axis regulation and modulate various brain circuitries' response to stress.[3]

Postinfectious IBS (PI-IBS) is another condition of stress-related changes in gastrointestinal functions that is driven by the interactions between psychosocial factors and local inflammation (see Chapter 18). The presence of significant life stressors occurring around the time of infection and related alteration in sympathetic modulation of immune function is reported to be one of the risk factors for developing PI-IBS, which occurs in 3% to 30% of individuals after acute gastroenteritis. Other risk factors include female gender and psychological characteristics such as anxiety, depression, neuroticism, and somatization, all of which contribute to the persistence of low-grade inflammation.[4]

Alterations in the bi-directional interactions between the central nervous system (CNS) and gut enteric nervous/immune systems are recognized to be part of the multifaceted pathophysiological mechanisms of IBS. Stress-induced disturbances at every level of the brain-gut axis can affect the regulation of intestinal function as well as perception and emotional response to visceral events. At the level of the CNS, the stress response is modulated by attention to the stressors, cognitive appraisal, mood state, and emotions. Functional brain imaging studies in IBS patients have provided evidence of an exaggerated activation of a vigilance network (the prefrontal cortex) and a failure in activation of regions involved in pain inhibition (the anterior cingulate cortex). Importantly, the cingulate cortex, a critical pain center, integrates autonomic and endocrine functions and is involved in recall of emotional experiences. At the ANS level, stress-related disturbances frequently occur in IBS patients. Those are characterized by decreased parasympathetic activity and increased sympathetic outflow, which impact on the neurally mediated regulation of colonic and immune function. Autonomic dysregulation may also account for many extra-intestinal symptoms occurring in IBS patients and the frequent overlap of IBS with other chronic pain disorders, such as fibromyalgia, migraine headache, chronic pelvic pain, and chronic fatigue syndrome. At the peripheral level of the brain-gut axis, stress-related modulation of the mucosal immune system and existing low-grade intestinal inflammation are increasingly recognized as contributing factors in the pathophysiology of functional gastrointestinal disorders. In particular, stress-induced activation and/or sensitization of mucosal mast cells play a pivotal role in the neuroimmune cross-talk involved in alterations in visceral sensitivity and increased intestinal permeability and bacterial translocation. Furthermore, in light of evidence of stress-related alterations of bacterial-host interaction, the potential role of probiotics in IBS treatment is gaining attention. Therefore, a concept of psychoneuroimmunology embraces the enteric neuroimmunological dysfunction in IBS as well as the influence of the central nervous system as a regulator of immunological response to stress.[2,4]

In recent years, the underlying biochemical coding of the stress response has been unraveled. Activation of the corticotropin releasing factor (CRF) signaling system (composed of peptides, CRF, and urocortins acting on two receptors—CRF_1 and/or CRF_2) has emerged as the primary pathway mediating the endocrine- and autonomic-related alterations of the immune system and gastrointestinal tract, as well as behavioral changes in rodents and non-human primates. There is compelling experimental evidence from animal studies that CRF_1 receptor activation in the brain and the colon plays a role in mediating stressors-related anxiogenic behavior, visceral hyperalgesia, increased colonic propulsive motor function, defecation, diarrhea, mucus secretion, mast cell activation, paracellular permeability, and proinflammatory response (Figure 15-1). The involvement of CRF_1 receptors in both the anxiogenic and colonic responses to stressors, a profile that is also observed in a subset of IBS patients, may be of relevance as an underlying mechanism for the coexistence of IBS and anxiety disorders, which is observed in up to 40% of IBS patients. Psychiatric disorders and various psychological disturbances do not seem to be directly connected with the occurrence of IBS, but they strongly influence symptom experience, individual illness behavior (eg, consultation pattern), and ultimately the treatment outcome.[5]

The modulatory role of either acute or chronic physical and psychological stressors in shaping the clinical course of IBS symptomatology and patients' quality of life is also supported by treatment modalities for IBS using complementary and alternative medicine practices intended to reduce stress perception that have resulted in encouraging outcome. Those include a broad range of evidence-based mind-body interventions like psychotherapy, cognitive-behavioral therapy, hypnotherapy, relaxation exercises, mindfulness meditation, as well as treatment with centrally targeted medications such as anxiolytics, selective serotonin reuptake inhibitors, and low doses of tricyclic antidepressants. The symptomatic improvement seems to be related to the modulation of the stress response, restoration of the ANS balance, and changes in the brain activation pattern in response to visceral stimuli.[6] In addition, owing to its well-characterized role in stress response, the CRF_1 system has been proposed as a relevant potential target for pharmacologic intervention using newly developed CRF_1 receptor antagonists, which are currently in phase II/III clinical trials for anxiety and IBS; however, no clear outcome has yet been reported.[7]

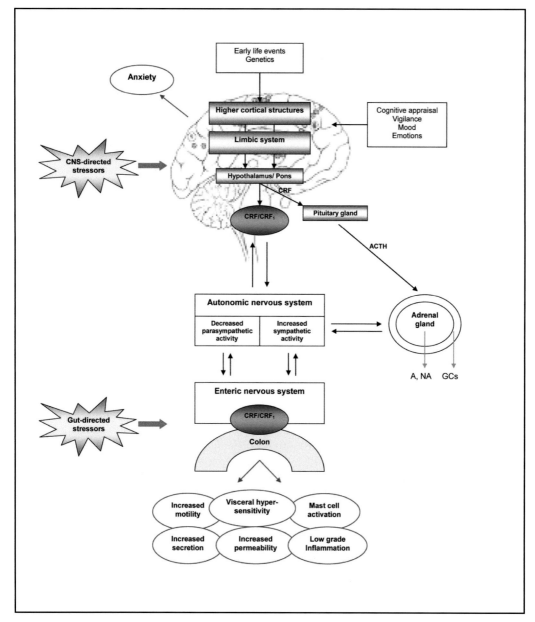

Figure 15-1. Activation of CRF$_1$ receptor signaling pathways in behavioral, neuroendocrine, and visceral response to CNS-directed (eg, psychological stress) and gut-directed (eg, infection) stressors based on preclinical evidence and pilot human studies.

A—adrenaline; ACTH—adrenocorticotropic hormone; CNS—central nervous system; CRF—corticotropin releasing factor; GCs—glucocorticoids; NA—noradrenaline.

References

1. Chrousos GR. Stress and disorders of the stress system. *Nat Rev Endocrinol.* 2009;5:374-381.
2. Mayer EA, Naliboff BD, Chang L, Coutinho SV. Stress and the gastrointestinal tract V. Stress and irritable bowel syndrome. *Am J Physiol Gastrointest Liver Physiol.* 2001;280:G519-G524.
3. Heitkemper M, Jarrett M. Irritable bowel syndrome: does gender matter? *J Psychosom Res.* 2008;64:583-587.
4. Spiller R, Garsed K. Infection, inflammation, and the irritable bowel syndrome. *Dig Liver Dis.* 2009;41: 844-849.
5. Taché Y, Brunnhuber S. From Hans Selye's discovery of biological stress to the identification of corticotropin-releasing factor signaling pathways: implication in stress-related functional bowel diseases. *Ann N Y Acad Sci.* 2008;1148:29-41.
6. Kearney DJ, Brown-Chang J. Complementary and alternative medicine for IBS in adults: mind-body interventions. *Nat Clin Pract Gastroenterol Hepatol.* 2008;5:624-636.
7. Zorrilla EP, Koob GF. Progess in corticotropin-releasing factor-1 antagonist development. *Drug Discov Today.* 2010;15:371-383.

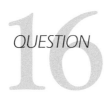

DOES ANXIETY OR DEPRESSION CAUSE IBS?

David A. Klibansky, MD and Kevin W. Olden, MD

A question that commonly arises among both clinicians and laypeople alike is the role psychiatric disorders play in the development of irritable bowel syndrome (IBS). Both psychologic distress and abdominal distress are common in the general US population and frequently coexist, but does this necessarily imply a causal relationship?

In the United States, recent surveys estimate lifetime prevalence for mood and anxiety disorders of approximately 21% and 30%, respectively. Similarly, irritable bowel syndrome is quite common and appears to affect anywhere from 6% to 20% of the US population, although only a small percentage of those affected ever present to a clinical provider for evaluation and management of their gastrointestinal (GI) symptoms (see Chapter 9). Interestingly, however, disorders such as depression and anxiety are disproportionately represented by people afflicted with IBS who are referred to GI providers, with a prevalence as high as 40% to 60% in some studies.[1]

Historically, there have been a number of theories regarding the relationship between psychiatric disorders and IBS, most of which have since been debunked. In the 1950s, psychoanalytic thinkers such as Alexander felt that IBS represented a defect in ego functioning with inadequate defense mechanisms.[2] Alexander and his contemporaries felt that only psychotherapy could manage the condition, referred to at the time as "colonic neurosis." In addition to psychotherapy, recommended management of the patient with severe symptoms included isolation in a hospital for complete rest, away from all family and business. Attitudes regarding the management of IBS are well characterized by the following quote: "The clinician to be universally successful in the management of these patients should possess the training of an internist and psychiatrist and the wisdom of a philosopher."[3]

Currently, our understanding of the potential causes of IBS has progressed significantly, although clearly many questions remain. Although the exact etiology of IBS remains elusive, there is significant clinical evidence demonstrating an interaction between multiple potential variables, including genetic predisposition, alterations in gastrointestinal motility, and abnormal sensation of normal gut physiology (otherwise known as visceral hypersensitivity). In addition, the state of knowledge as to the relationship between psychosocial factors and organic disease in general has progressed tremendously. One significant paradigm shift involves the adaptation of the "biopsychosocial model" as advocated by Engel. This approach values the reciprocal interaction between the brain and the gut. That is to say, primary psychological processes may modify GI physiology, and conversely GI dysfunction may alter neurologic and psychologic processing. There are, in fact, a number of ways through which psychological factors may influence symptoms of IBS. Psychological distress may lower gastrointestinal symptom thresholds mediated by the central nervous system, directly alter GI motility and physiology through the brain-gut axis, or result in altered attitudes or thought processes regarding existing IBS symptoms.[1,4] Moreover, there is significant overlap in the neurochemical signaling pathways between the central and enteric nervous systems. Indeed, it has been demonstrated that medications traditionally used for the treatment of mood disorders (such as tricyclic antidepressants), even when used at doses much lower than is necessary for management of depression or anxiety, improve symptoms of IBS. This effect may relate to the modulation of similar neurochemical pathways between the brain and GI tract. Conversely, clinical studies have shown that, for people with untreated anxiety or mood disorders who also have IBS, management of the psychologic disorder frequently results in more significant improvement in IBS symptoms than usual medical therapies targeted solely at the GI symptoms.[1,4]

Stress and Symptom Perception and Expression

It is not a secret that, for many patients, IBS symptoms can at times be disabling and significantly interfere with quality of life. The presence of psychiatric disorders or the presence of excessive stress has been demonstrated to alter pain thresholds for experimentally induced colonic distention with an inflatable balloon.[5] Similar research has demonstrated that people with anxiety or mood disorders are more likely to experience significant distress from their symptoms, rate their pain as more severe, and seek out medical care with heightened concern about a serious underlying illness such as cancer. It is not clear whether a perception of increased symptom severity is the result of a chronic state of symptom amplification mediated by the central nervous system or more local changes occurring at the level of the GI tract. Regardless, it is clear that these symptoms are significant to the affected person and can be debilitating, often to a degree greater than symptoms related to structural GI pathology, such as peptic ulcer disease or chronic liver disease.[6]

The Issue of Abuse

In the past 20 years, a number of studies have demonstrated a much higher rate of prior sexual, physical, or emotional abuse in patients with IBS or IBS-related illness. It is known that stressful life events are associated with symptom exacerbation in IBS, and prior abuse may be related to mood disorders or post-traumatic stress disorder (PTSD). This in turn can result in elevated chronic life stress, which in turn can generate serious psychological symptoms and poor illness coping.[5,7] To this regard, an underlying psychiatric disorder that has resulted from prior abuse may function as a mediator of more severe and poorly tolerated symptoms.

Despite the increased frequency of mood and anxiety disorders among people with IBS referred to a GI provider, it is notable that no psychological studies have ever demonstrated a consistent psychological profile or personality type among people with IBS. Studies such as these are quite important as they demonstrate that IBS is a unique disease unto itself and that there is no single underlying psychologic predisposition. What studies do appear to demonstrate is that the presence of anxiety or mood disorders in those who happen to develop IBS may result in more severe or poorly tolerated symptoms through the previously mentioned mechanisms. Given the potential for frequent pain and discomfort, it may be questioned whether anxiety and depression may in fact develop as a consequence of severe IBS, rather than exist as a modifier. Although clearly there is potential for a self-propagating viscous cycle between anxiety or mood symptoms and IBS symptoms, in the majority of cases, mood and anxiety disorders predate or present simultaneously with severe IBS, rather than after.

Given the relationships above, it becomes clear that although neither anxiety nor depression are thought to directly cause IBS, they are present with high frequency in those with IBS, particularly in people with more severe symptoms requiring referral to a GI office. As stated, there is evidence that these disorders may directly influence IBS symptoms even if they do not represent a primary cause. Because of this, it would seem apparent that a multimodal approach to the management of IBS is most likely to result in a successful outcome. This includes screening for any conditions such as anxiety and depression or any prior history of abuse with plan for appropriate management or referral for these conditions if identified. It should be stressed to the patient that this does not imply that GI symptoms are "made up" or the direct result of an underlying psychiatric disorder. Rather, it should be understood that the brain and gut are intimately connected, and, even if not evident to the afflicted person, both may intimately affect the other. Given this, management of all aspects of patient care including medical, social, and psychiatric conditions is imperative for the patient with IBS. Failure to do so is likely to result in poorly controlled symptoms with resultant ongoing frustration for both the patient and provider alike. Successful engagement of the patient in a treatment program that addresses all aspects of their care, including psychosocial issues, has the potential to afford superior symptomatic relief and yield a rewarding patient-clinician interaction.

References

1. Levy RL, Olden KW, Naliboff BD, et al. Psychosocial aspects of the functional gastrointestinal disorders. *Gastroenterology*. 2006;130:1447-1458.
2. Olden KW. Irritable bowel syndrome: what is the role of the psyche? *Digest Liver Dis*. 2006;38:200-201.
3. Bockus HL. *Gastroenterology*. Philadelphia: W.B. Saunders;1944:475-533.
4. Budavari AI, Olden KW. Psychosocial aspects of functional gastrointestinal disorders. *Gastroenterol Clin N Am*. 2003;32:477-506.
5. Ritchie J. Pain from distention of pelvic colon by inflating a balloon in the irritable bowel syndrome. *Gut*. 1973;6:105-112.

6. Drossman DA, Li Z, Leseman J. Health status by gastrointestinal diagnosis and abuse history. *Gastroenterology.* 1996;110:999-1007.
7. Drossman DA, Talley NJ, Leserman J, Olden KW, Barreiro MA. Sexual and physical abuse and gastrointestinal illness. *Ann Intern Med.* 1995;123:782-794.

IBS AND THE MENSTRUAL CYCLE: WHAT IS THE RELATIONSHIP?

Lin Chang, MD and Margaret M. Heitkemper, PhD, RN, FAAN

Population studies have shown that the occurrence of irritable bowel syndrome (IBS) is related to gender and age. In Western cultures, IBS has a female predominance with a female-to-male ratio of 2 to 2.5:1 in those who seek health care. However, Eastern population studies report equal or slightly higher female-to-male ratio in the prevalence of IBS, which suggests that cultural differences may also play a role in IBS symptom reporting. Studies have demonstrated that female gender is a significant independent risk factor for new-onset IBS and postinfectious IBS. In both the general population and IBS patient population, women report more gastrointestinal (GI) and non-GI symptoms than men.

Clinical and biological evidence regarding gender and gender-related differences relevant to IBS has led to the hypothesis that ovarian hormone levels may result in a greater vulnerability of women to develop IBS.[1] Most women with IBS who seek health care are of reproductive age. Furthermore, studies have shown that both the prevalence and incidence of IBS in women declines after the age of 40 years, while they remain relatively stable, albeit lower, in men. Both women with and without IBS report increased IBS symptoms at the onset of menses, although symptom severity is higher in women with IBS than healthy women. Studies have reported sex and gender differences in colorectal sensory perception, colonic motility, colonic mucosal mast cell count, brain activation patterns to visceral stimulation, and treatment response to certain IBS therapies. There are only limited data on the effect of hormonal therapy and menopause in IBS. This chapter will address key points related to the effect of the menstrual cycle on IBS symptoms and gut function.

Are There Gender Differences in IBS Symptoms?

A recent meta-analysis and systematic review was performed to assess gender differences in individual IBS symptoms in the general and IBS patient populations.[2] In the general population, women were more likely to report abdominal pain and pain-related IBS diagnostic symptoms, although this gender difference was not present in the IBS patient population. Compared to men, women were more likely to report the supportive symptoms of IBS, particularly constipation-related symptoms such as bloating, distension, and straining. Similarly, in IBS patients, women demonstrated a considerably higher risk for constipation-related symptoms including abdominal distension, bloating, infrequent stools, and hard stools than men with IBS. Men with IBS were significantly more likely to report the diarrhea-related symptoms of loose/watery stools and increased stool frequency than women with IBS. These gender differences in IBS symptoms were reported in both Western and Eastern studies.

The generally higher IBS symptom reporting in women compared to men may be due to several reasons. Women typically seek more healthcare visits and have greater symptom recall than do men. In addition, gender and sex-related differences have been demonstrated in GI function, including transit time, visceral perception, and brain activation patterns to visceral sensory stimuli, which can conceivably contribute to the greater prevalence of IBS symptoms in women and the gender differences in bowel habits.

What Effect Does the Menstrual Cycle Have on IBS Symptoms?

The severity of GI symptoms, including abdominal pain, altered bowel habits, and bloating, varies across phases of the menstrual cycle. Not all women with IBS report an association between cycle phase and symptoms. Although there are methodologic differences between studies that assessed the effect of menstrual cycle on IBS symptoms, the majority of studies report increased GI symptoms at the time of menses compared to other phases. Abdominal discomfort and pain symptoms have been reported at premenses (days immediately preceding the onset of menses) and menses in women ages 19 to 37 years, when compared with other cycle phases. In particular, increases in loose stools and bloating have been reported at the time of menses in most studies. Increased abdominal pain and changes in stool frequency are less commonly reported.[1]

What Effect Does the Menstrual Cycle Have on Gut Function as it Pertains to IBS?

Exacerbations of a number of medical conditions including IBS are linked with phases of the menstrual cycle.[3] Migraines, headaches, asthma, as well as psychological distress have all been found to be more prevalent in women with these conditions around the time of menses (mid-late luteal, premenses, and menses phases). In addition, women with IBS are more likely to report dysmenorrhea and premenstrual distress than women without IBS. Given the natural fluctuations in ovarian hormones (estrogen and progesterone) that occur across the menstrual cycle, it is not difficult to imagine that these exacerbations are hormonally driven. In particular, the subsequent drop in both progesterone and estrogen levels following their ovulation-induced rise during the luteal phase may set the stage for neurochemical, blood flow, motility, and pain sensitivity changes in susceptible women prior to the onset of menses.

What Effects Do Ovarian Hormones Have on IBS Symptoms?

The gonadal hormones (estrogen and progesterone) may influence visceral pain and discomfort sensations between the gastrointestinal organs and the brain.[1] The interactions among estrogen and progesterone and pathways responsible for pain transmission are complex and occur at multiple levels. For example, estrogen has been shown to have both pain facilitory and inhibitory effects on afferent sensory as well as central modulatory neurons. Both estrogen and progesterone have been found to have receptors on gastrointestinal tract smooth muscle. Because of the range and multiplicity of these effects, determination of the mechanisms underlying ovarian hormonal influence on pain perception or neural activity has been difficult.

It has been suggested that oral contraceptives modestly reduce but do not eliminate GI symptoms in women with IBS. However, there has been little study of the effects of these agents in IBS. Dysmenorrhea, which often co-occurs in women with IBS, is alleviated by the use of oral contraceptives.

What Is the Effect of Menopause on IBS?

Only a handful of studies have compared the presence of IBS symptoms in premenopausal versus postmenopausal women, and most are retrospective. In women with IBS, nausea was the only symptom reported more frequently by premenopausal women than postmenopausal women. In a recent, prospective study by Cain and colleagues, postmenopausal women with IBS reported more abdominal bloating and distension and somatic pain symptoms than premenopausal women with IBS, although these differences did not maintain statistical significance after controlling for age.[4] Among healthy women, gaseousness and excessive flatulence were the only GI symptoms that were significantly more prevalent in postmenopausal women. Few data are available to determine whether hormone replacement therapy has an effect on IBS symptoms in postmenopausal women.

Summary

Existing literature supports the presence of overall gender differences in the prevalence of IBS and individual IBS symptoms, although these differences are modest. Women are more likely to report symptoms associated with constipation, particularly bloating and distension. Bloating and distension are also more frequently reported at the onset of menses compared to other menstrual cycle phases and by postmenopausal women with IBS compared to premenopausal women. Preclinical and clinical studies suggest that estrogen and progesterone can affect brain-gut pathways involved in pain sensitivity and GI function, although these mechanisms are complex. Animal research studies support an enhancing effect of estrogen and progesterone on visceral sensitivity, particularly under stress conditions. Their effects are less clear in human studies as data are very limited. Larger, well-designed studies that are focused on assessing the role of ovarian hormones on IBS symptoms and the effect of menopausal status in IBS are needed. In clinical practice, the key points to keep in mind are that women are more likely than men to report constipation-associated symptoms than men, GI and non-GI symptoms can increase in some women with IBS during the premenses period, but it is not clear if oral contraceptives decrease these cyclical changes, and little is known about the effect of menopause or hormone replacement therapy on IBS symptoms.

References

1. Heitkemper MM, Chang L. Do fluctuations in ovarian hormones affect gastrointestinal symptoms in women with irritable bowel syndrome? *Gend Med.* 2009;6(Suppl 2):152-167.
2. Adeyemo M, Spiegel BMS, Chang L. Systematic analysis of gender-related differences in irritable bowel syndrome (IBS) symptoms. *Aliment Pharmacol Ther.* 2010;32(6):738-755.
3. Heitkemper MM, Jarrett M. Pattern of gastrointestinal and somatic symptoms across the menstrual cycle. *Gastroenterology.* 1992;102:505-513.
4. Cain KC, Jarrett ME, Burr RL, Rosen S, Hertig VL, Heitkemper MM. Gender differences in gastrointestinal, psychological, and somatic symptoms in irritable bowel syndrome. *Dig Dis Sci.* 2009;54:1542-1549.

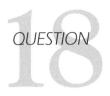
HOW DOES AN INFECTION CAUSE IBS?

Kok-Ann Gwee, FRCP, PhD

In as many as 25% of all irritable bowel syndrome (IBS) patients, an episode of infectious diarrhea may precede the onset of persistent bowel disturbances. In these patients with postinfectious IBS (PI-IBS), symptoms usually take the form of recurrent abdominal pain and diarrhea. The risk of developing IBS after a prior infection ranged from 4% in the community to 26% in patients with a severe infection requiring hospitalization. Bacterial infections with *Salmonella, Campylobacter,* and *Shigella* were most consistently implicated. It appears that PI-IBS arises from the convergence of biological and psychological factors.

When patients with acute gastroenteritis were followed prospectively, the patients who developed IBS had a longer duration of an acute diarrheal illness. Rectal biopsies taken at the time of the acute illness also suggest that these patients could have had more severe inflammation as evidenced by enhanced mucosal expression of the pro-inflammatory cytokine interleukin 1β m RNA.[1] In the period following recovery from the acute infection, there is evidence in PI-IBS of persistent immune activation, such as intra-epithelial lymphocytosis and enhanced mucosal IL-1β m RNA expression in rectal biopsies.[1,2]

On the other hand, in our study, we found that psychological traits, such as hypochondriasis, somatization, neuroticism, and anxiety, were predictors of who might develop IBS postinfection.[3] Our most significant finding was that patients who developed IBS after an infection were more likely to have experienced psychologically traumatic life events preceding their infection than those who recovered without IBS. Furthermore, during the 3 months after the infection, PI-IBS patients continued to report more stressful life events.

When studies were carried out at 3 months postinfection, the following physiological disturbances were observed—rapid whole gut transit times, lower threshold for pain and increased rectal contractility in response to rectal distension, reduced rectal compliance, and increased intestinal permeability.[2,3] These disturbances were observed even in patients who had recovered from the infection without IBS sequelae but were more severe in patients who developed PI-IBS.

We believe that these functional disturbances were due to the infection and the associated inflammation. This is supported by a series of studies employing a mouse model of postinfective gut dysfunction.[4] In these studies, experimental mice were infected with the nematode *Trichinella spiralis* by gavage. To study intestinal neuromuscular function during and after recovery from acute intestinal inflammation, longitudinal muscle strips were obtained from the jejunum, and smooth muscle contractility responses to cholinergic and electrical field stimulation of intramural nerves were measured. Inflammatory activity and immune activation were measured by various cellular, enzymatic, and molecular markers and were found to correlate with neuromuscular dysfunction. Furthermore, other similar animal models have also demonstrated that experimental stress can enhance the response to inflammatory stimulus and subsequently reactivate quiescent colitis.

Putting all these data together, we have proposed a biopsychosocial model of post-infectious IBS. We believe that an episode of infectious diarrhea may produce changes in gastrointestinal physiology that predispose to symptoms of diarrhea and abdominal pain. Psychosocial factors such as stress and personality would influence the immune response and, thus, modulate the severity of inflammatory-mediated changes in neuro-muscular function of the gastrointestinal tract. At a psychosomatic level, we believe that the occurrence of infection at a stressful time creates a long-lived association between stressful situations and bowel symptoms, such that future stressful events may precipitate physiological disturbances in the gastrointestinal tract reminiscent of the index infectious event.

References

1. Gwee KA, Collins SM, Read NW, et al. Increased rectal mucosal expression of interleukin 1B in recently acquired post-infectious irritable bowel syndrome. *Gut.* 2003;52:523-526.
2. Spiller RC, Jenkins D, Thornley JP, et al. Increased rectal mucosal enteroendocrine cells, T lymphocytes and increased gut permeability following acute *Campylobacter enteritis* and in post-dysenteric irritable bowel syndrome. *Gut.* 2000;47:804-811.
3. Gwee KA, Leong YL, Graham C, et al. The role of psychological and biological factors in postinfective gut dysfunction. *Gut.* 1999;44:400-406.
4. Barbara G, Vallance BA, Collins SM. Persistent intestinal neuromuscular dysfunction after acute nematode infection in mice. *Gastroenterology.* 1997;113:1224-1232.

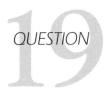

IS THERE A RELATIONSHIP BETWEEN SURGERY AND IBS?

Ami D. Sperber, MD, MSPH

I find the question of a possible association between surgery and irritable bowel syndrome (IBS) intriguing in relation to both my clinical practice and research. It is a relevant issue for doctors in disciplines as varied as family medicine, gastroenterology, general surgery, and gynecology. Over the years, I have treated many IBS patients who had previously undergone abdominal or pelvic surgeries, such as appendectomy, cholecystectomy, and hysterectomy. In many of these cases, the symptoms that led to the decision to operate persisted after surgery, and the clinical course was either unaltered or got worse.

Actually, there are 2 related, but different, issues of interest. The first is whether surgery can lead to the development IBS. The second is whether there is an association between surgery and IBS regardless of temporality (ie, is there evidence of cause and effect?).

Can abdominal or pelvic surgery cause IBS? Unfortunately, there is little available information to answer this question. However, posing the question makes sense. Research on the pathophysiology of IBS, as well as other painful functional GI disorders, has focused on visceral hypersensitivity (ie, lower sensory thresholds to bowel distension and dysregulation of brain-gut interactions at higher levels of the enteric and central nervous systems). Visceral hypersensitivity can stem from, among other causes, locally injurious factors to the intestinal tract, including bacterial infection or direct injury to the bowel, for example, by surgery. This may then lead to inflammation and/or sensitization of visceral afferent nerves. In addition, brain-gut dysregulation may manifest as central enhancement of incoming visceral signals that could be modulated by chronic stress, impaired coping skills, psychological distress, and psychiatric comorbidity, all of which may lead to increased pain reporting. Thus, brain-gut dysregulation, regardless of the level of the brain-gut axis at which it takes place, could be initiated by a precipitating event such as abdominal or pelvic surgery. Theoretically, IBS or chronic pain could result from surgical "insult" either by way of direct local surgical injury or due to central amplification related to psychosocial distress.

To answer these questions, we need prospective, controlled studies with large study populations. My coinvestigators and I conducted a prospective, controlled study on 123 women undergoing elective gynecologic surgery for non-pain indications who were then followed for 1 year postoperatively, in parallel with a matched control group of 132 women who visited gynecology clinics for non-pain reasons and did not have surgery.[1] The results of this study showed that three women who did not have any symptoms of IBS prior to surgery fulfilled the Rome II diagnostic criteria for IBS at postoperative follow-up, compared with none in the control group. This finding did not reach statistical significance, most likely because the study was underpowered to answer this question and possibly because the Rome II criteria are fairly restrictive, leading to lower rates of diagnosis than the currently used Rome III criteria. However, our results do provide justification for further investigation of this question.

Our study did have 2 statistically significant findings. The first was that significantly more patients (15.3%) in the surgery group developed abdominal pain at follow-up than the control group (3.6%; $P=0.003$). The second was that hysterectomy does not cause subsequent constipation, in contrast to the results of previously reported, but uncontrolled, studies.[2] The predictive analysis showed that a number of psychosocial variables, specifically anticipation of difficult recovery from the operation, low coping skills, perceived severity of the illness, and personal controllability, predicted the development of abdominal pain. In contrast, the socio-demographic, biologic, and surgery-related variables did not predict the development of postoperative abdominal pain. The study findings hint at the possibility that psychosocial variables related to individual patient characteristics may have the greatest effect, highlighting the potential etiological importance of central amplification of visceral signals.

At present, there is no definitive answer to the first question as to whether abdominal or pelvic surgery can cause IBS, but there is evidence suggestive of a possible cause and effect relationship between abdominal or pelvic surgery and the development of chronic abdominal pain or even IBS. Obviously, further studies are needed to strengthen or challenge these hypotheses. The resulting information could be of value in the future for the development of patient-centered treatment strategies aimed at pre-empting the development of postsurgical abdominal pain or IBS.

Is there an association between surgery and IBS regardless of temporality (cause and effect)? In contrast to the first question, there is a substantial body of information in the medical literature on this second question. As early as 1928, a paper was published in the *Lancet* reporting a high rate of appendectomy in patients with "chronic spasmodic affectations of the colon," while later reports described a relatively high rate of appendectomies without evidence of appendicitis.

The most comprehensive studies to date have been conducted among HMO members or examinees. A study of 89,008 examinees in the Kaiser Permanente Medical Care Plan in the San Diego region, of whom 5.2% were diagnosed with IBS, compared examinees with and without IBS for a history of previous abdominal/pelvic surgery. Strong independent associations with IBS were found for cholecystectomy (12.4% versus 4.1%, respectively, $P<0.0001$), appendectomy (21.1% versus 11.7%; $P<0.0001$), and hysterectomy (33.2% versus 17.0%; $P<0.0001$).[3] The adjusted odds ratios for cholecystectomy, appendectomy, and hysterectomy, respectively, were 2.09, 1.45, and 1.70. Other studies have reported similar trends. While IBS patients have higher rates of cholecystectomy, there is no evidence that they have higher rates of cholelithiasis.

Why are the rates of these surgeries so high among IBS patients? Setting aside the questions of whether surgery can cause IBS, the most widely proposed explanation is misdiagnosis. As we know from clinical experience, many patients with IBS, especially those with greater symptom severity, have high rates of comorbid nongastrointestinal pain conditions, such as fibromyalgia, and high rates of psychological comorbidity, including anxiety and somatization. These patients are characterized by a high rate of doctor visits ("doctor shopping") and emergency room visits. They often are very demanding in their encounters with us. Over time, it is more and more likely that one of these encounters will lead a treating doctor to suspect cholecystitis, appendicitis, or a gynecological disorder enough that laparoscopy or even open surgery is felt to be indicated. As mentioned earlier, in many of these cases, the symptoms that led to the decision to operate persist after surgery, and the clinical course is either unaltered or gets worse.

The bottom line is that IBS patients undergo significantly more surgeries, such as cholecystectomy, hysterectomy, and appendectomy, than control groups, in many cases without appropriate indications. While the reasons for this have not been completely determined, some of these operations could be averted with a higher level of awareness of the presentation of IBS and its psychosocial aspects among nongastroenterology specialists and with a greater degree of clinical cooperation among family physicians, general surgeons, gynecologists, and gastroenterologists.

One way to do this is to initiate collaborative clinics to review and discuss cases of mutual interest. I have participated, to my great benefit, in multidisciplinary staff meetings where cases in which surgery was being considered were presented and discussed in terms of the indications and differential diagnosis. We have also reviewed in these meetings the cases of patients who already had surgery, without surgical or histological evidence of the disease for which they were referred. Review sessions of this type can increase clinical awareness and, perhaps, reduce the number of unnecessary future operations.

Other opportunities to reduce unnecessary surgery include a greater frequency of consultations between gynecologists, surgeons, and gastroenterologists, more involvement in the decision process of family physicians who have greater knowledge of their patients' psychosocial issues (this is not the case in many parts of the world), and multidisciplinary continuing education programs in which these issues can be raised and discussed.

Summary

Further research can help clarify the first question as to whether abdominal or pelvic surgery can cause IBS. Assuming that we know that IBS is associated with surgery, a variety of multidisciplinary clinical strategies can help reduce the extent of inappropriate surgery among IBS patients.

References

1. Sperber AD, Blank Morris C, Greemberg L, et al. Development of abdominal pain and IBS following gynecological surgery: a prospective, controlled study. *Gastroenterology.* 2008;134:75-84.
2. Sperber AD, Blank Morris C, Greemberg L, et al. Constipation does not develop following elective hysterectomy: a prospective, controlled study. *Neurogastroenterol Motil.* 2009;21:18-22.
3. Longstreth GF, Yao JF. Irritable bowel syndrome and surgery: a multivariable analysis. *Gastroenterology.* 2004;126:1665-1673.

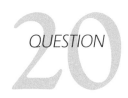
Is There an Association Between IBS and IBD?

L. Campbell Levy, MD, and Corey A. Siegel, MD

Despite considerable overlap between symptoms of irritable bowel syndrome (IBS) and inflammatory bowel disease (IBD), these disorders are regarded as separate entities with distinct diagnostic criteria and pathophysiologic underpinnings. However, the boundaries separating these 2 disorders have recently become somewhat blurred. Microscopic inflammation has been implicated in the pathogenesis of IBS, while subsets of IBD patients exhibit symptoms disproportionate to disease activity and more consistent with IBS. Investigating the role of microscopic inflammation and visceral pain may lead to future novel therapies for both of these common diseases. More pertinent to clinical practice, it remains a formidable and important challenge to accurately identify these processes in order to avoid mislabeling patients, which can delay diagnosis, lead to undertreatment or inappropriate treatments, and expose patients to futile, potentially harmful, and expensive therapies.

Prevalence of IBS in IBD

Bloating, diarrhea, abdominal pain, and incontinence are common among patients with IBD during times of active inflammation but also during times of minimal or absent gross mucosal inflammation. Approximately 20% of IBD patients in clinical and endoscopic remission continue to experience IBS-like symptoms.[1] Based on the epidemiology of IBS and IBD, the coexistence of these disorders is not surprising. The prevalence of IBD is 0.1% to 0.2%, which is dwarfed by the prevalence of IBS (approximately 15%). Therefore, one would expect that 10% to 20% of IBD patients would also have IBS, although IBS-type symptoms appear to be even more common among individuals with IBD.[2]

Data from two separate cross-sectional studies demonstrate that, among patients with ulcerative colitis (UC) and Crohn's disease (CD) who were in remission, 33% and 42% to 57% respectively suffered from IBS-like symptoms.[3] Criticisms of these data have included the reliance on symptom scores that can overlap with functional syndromes and the lack of objective investigations to identify active inflammation. A more recent study examined fecal calprotectin as a surrogate marker for disease activity to differentiate functional symptoms from those of ongoing occult inflammation. Sixty percent of patients with CD disease and 40% of patients with UC fulfilled Rome II criteria for IBS. Fecal calprotectin was significantly higher in the IBD patients with IBS symptoms compared to those patients without IBS-type symptoms (for CD patients: 414.7 versus 174.9, $P=0.009$; for UC patients: 591.1 versus 229.8, $P=0.004$).[3] A similar study in a cohort of IBD patients from the United Kingdom found that, after excluding patients with elevated fecal calprotectin, the rate of IBS resembled that of the general population. Together, these data suggest that IBS symptoms in IBD patients may reflect active inflammation, and an elevated CRP can help to identify those in which better IBD-directed therapy is necessary.

Visceral Hypersensitivity and Dysmotility in IBD

Apart from the prevalence of IBS among IBD patients, there is evidence to suggest that abnormal motility and visceral hypersensitivity play a role in the development of functional symptoms in IBD patients. In UC patients, both abnormal basal contractile activity of the distal colon and persistently increased small bowel motility, in the absence of active disease, have been described.[2] When compared to both healthy controls and to patients with colitis in remission, individuals with active UC have lower colonic sensory thresholds. Autonomic and sensory neuropathies unexplained by nutritional deficiencies or medications may occur in IBD patients, which suggests that demyelination or small fiber neuropathy may be a manifestation of IBD. Experimental animal data support the idea that persistent or previously resolved inflammation may result in visceral hyperalgesia due in part to increased neuronal excitability.[1]

Postinfectious IBS, Low-Grade Inflammation, and Immune Dysregulation

First described in 1962 by Chaudary and Truelove, the concept of postinfectious irritable bowel syndrome (PI-IBS) blurs the artificial and mutually exclusive concept of a patient having either functional hypersensitivity or chronic inflammation. It has been estimated that PI-IBS follows a bacterial or viral infection in up to 36% of individuals.[4] The risk of developing IBS as a sequelae of an acute infectious gastroenteritis was estimated at sevenfold (OR 7.3, 95% CI 4.7 to 11.1) that of controls in a meta-analysis of eight studies.[5] Because infection has also been implicated as a possible trigger for IBD (by instigating an inappropriate immune response that leads to chronic mucosal inflammation), new-onset Crohn's disease or UC should also be considered in the differential diagnosis when IBS-like symptoms persist after an acute gastrointestinal infection.[6]

Colonoscopy studies demonstrated that patients with PI-IBS have longstanding changes of chronic inflammation, albeit microscopic or "low grade." After the body has "cleared" the infectious agent, biopsies show a persistence of CD3 and CD8 T lymphocytes and increased expression of interleukin-1β in colonic biopsies. Ileal biopsies have shown increased mast cells, which may increase gut permeability. Increased permeability potentially initiates chronic inflammation via increased translocation of bacterial antigens similar to mechanisms thought to be essential in the development of IBD.[2]

Similar signals of immune dysregulation have been detected in the mucosa and blood of subgroups of IBS patients. An inappropriately activated adaptive immune response has been implicated in the pathogenesis of IBS due to increased numbers of $CD4^+$ and $CD8^+$ T cells found within the intestinal mucosa. Increased innate immune activity has been detected in patients with IBS irrespective of bowel habit pattern, as compared to healthy controls. There are increased numbers of mast cells within the cecum and increased secretion of the proinflammatory cytokines IL-6, IL-1β, and TNF from mononuclear cells.[4] In fact, altered secretion of inflammatory cytokines and chemokines in IBS have led to the recent development of a commercially available diagnostic blood test for IBS. Prometheus IBS Diagnostic measures 10 serum markers applied in an algorithm designed to differentiate IBS from non-IBS. Four of the markers (tissue transglutaminase antibody, anti-*Saccharomyces cerevisiae* antibody, anti-Cbir1 antibody, and antineutrophil cytoplasmic antibody) have long been associated with chronic inflammatory conditions, such as celiac disease and IBD. Other markers in the panel, such as IL-1β and growth-related oncogene-α (GRO-α), play a central role in the inflammatory response and in the activation of neutrophils.[7]

Stress, Psychosocial Factors, and Neuroimmune Interactions

Mucosal inflammation and immune dysregulation may not be sufficient to explain the hyperalgesia and dysmotility seen in IBS patients and IBD patients who are in remission. Psychosocial factors, stress, and psychiatric disorders likely also play a crucial role in many patients. These factors have been associated with the generation and perpetuation of IBS symptoms. A large proportion of IBS patients referred for gastroenterology evaluation have comorbid psychiatric conditions.[8] Psychiatric conditions also frequently coexist with IBD and have been associated with the persistence of symptoms in patients who are otherwise in clinical remission. Moreover, psychological stress appears to be a necessary component for the development of PI-IBS. In one of the original studies of PI-IBS, psychological distress at the time of infection and persistent inflammation several months after infection were the major predictors of persistent symptoms[2] (see Chapter 18).

The impact of psychological stressors and alterations of central nervous regulatory systems on end-organ development of visceral symptoms is complex. Stimulation of corticotropin-releasing factor (CRF), an important mediator of central stress response, and dysfunction of the hypothalamus-pituitary-adrenal (HPA) axis may play a key role in the pathogenesis of symptoms in some IBS and IBD patients, although this needs further study.[2] Not only is centrally mediated neuroimmune dysfunction important, but there are data underscoring the importance of interactions with nerves and immune processes at the end-organ level. Several studies have shown increased densities of nerve fibers clustering around mast cells in PI-IBS, and in animal models of IBS, increased mast cells have been shown to excite visceral sensory neurons.[4]

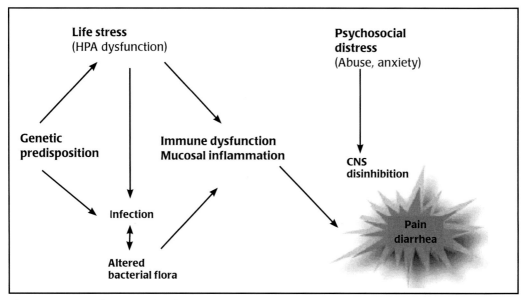

Figure 20-1. Unifying model for PI-IBS and IBD-IBS. A common genetic predisposition may contribute to immune dysfunction and chronic low-grade mucosal inflammation as a result of dysbiosis. This can result in IBS-type symptoms often in the setting of a significant psychosocial stressor. (Adapted from Grover M, Herfarth H, Drossman DA. The functional-organic dichotomy: postinfectious irritable bowel syndrome and inflammatory bowel disease-irritable bowel syndrome. *Clin Gastroenterol Hepatol.* 2009;7(1):48-53.)

IBS-IBD Model

There appear to be subsets of patients with IBD and IBS who both have chronic low-grade intestinal inflammation and who share many of the same attributes. Some investigators have unified the previously dualistic concept of IBS or IBD and describe it as an IBD-IBS model.[2] There may be a common genetic predisposition as has been described in Crohn's disease. In response to a stress—either centrally via hypothalamic-pituitary axis (HPA) dysfunction or locally via infection—the model proposes a resultant immune dysregulation and chronic low-grade inflammatory state. These factors eventually produce visceral pain and dysmotility, resulting potentially in multiple intestinal functional symptoms (Figure 20-1). The advantages of embracing such a model may be to avoid mislabeling patients as "refractory IBD" and to prevent escalating therapy with potentially harmful drugs that are likely to be futile. Furthermore, it offers a research and clinical framework on which to build and ask questions.

Practical Approach to Functional Intestinal Symptoms in IBD

Chronic functional abdominal symptoms, especially pain, can be frustrating for the patient and the clinician alike, and even worse, it can confound medical decision making. While the model of the IBD-IBS patient is provocative, it does not apply to every patient.

Table 20-1

Foods and Beverages That Might Aggravate IBS in IBD Patients[9]

Beverages	*Foods*	*Additives*
Milk	Anything containing dairy	Spices and seasoning
Caffeine-containing drinks	Fast food or Chinese food	Gravy, heavy sauces
Diet drinks	Fried or fatty foods	Artificial flavorings
Fruit juices	Whole or multigrain breads	Artificial sweeteners
Alcohol	Salads (plain lettuce OK)	Large amounts of fructose
	Beans and popcorn	
	Red meat	
	Cookies, cakes, and pies	

Therefore, because of the overlap of symptoms, it is critical to ascertain the degree of disease activity in patients with chronic IBD and IBS-like symptoms. This often requires both upper and lower endoscopy, as well as small bowel imaging. If these tests fail to reveal any evidence of active disease, then careful evaluation for other clinically pertinent causes of abdominal pain, such as abdominal wall pain or even rarely adrenal insufficiency, may be warranted.

For patients whose evaluation is otherwise unrevealing and who meet Rome III criteria, there is a significant likelihood that they fit within the IBS-IBD model. Gastroenterologists should screen these patients for coexisting psychiatric diagnoses and possible substance abuse and, when there is a concern, refer patients accordingly. For abdominal cramping and pain, we often use low-dose tricyclic antidepressants at our center, albeit with limited data and mixed responses. Food intolerances often coexist with IBS and IBD, and, therefore, in selected patients with cramping and a tendency to diarrhea, a food avoidance diet low in fiber, lactose, fructose, and fat can be helpful.[9] Dietary office-based counseling as well as distributing a list of foods to minimize or avoid gives patients some guidance to help identify whether certain elements in their diet are contributing to symptoms (Table 20-1). Behavioral treatments such as cognitive behavioral therapy and hypnosis have been used with success in IBS and may also benefit this subgroup of IBD patients.[2]

Summary

Current evidence indicates that the pathogenesis of functional intestinal symptoms are due to a complex interaction between the sensitizing effects of inflammation, immune dysregulation, and neuroimmune influences, which may be affected by emotional and psychosocial stressors. Better understanding of this biopsychosocial model may yield new therapeutic options in the future, but in the meantime, this subgroup of patients remains challenging to manage. Appreciating the overlap physiologically and clinically between IBS and IBD enables better identification of these patients, avoids inappropriate use of potentially harmful medications, and allows for a practical approach to a problem that may improve both patient and physician satisfaction.

References

1. Bielefeldt K, Davis B, Binion DG. Pain and inflammatory bowel disease. *Inflamm Bowel Dis.* 2009;15: 778-788.
2. Grover M, Herfarth H, Drossman DA. The functional-organic dichotomy: postinfectious irritable bowel syndrome and inflammatory bowel disease-irritable bowel syndrome. *Clin Gastroenterol Hepatol.* 2009;7:48-53.
3. Keohane J, O'Mahony C, O'Mahony L, O'Mahony S, Quigley EM, Shanahan F. Irritable bowel syndrome-type symptoms in patients with inflammatory bowel disease: a real association or reflection of occult inflammation? *Am J Gastroenterol.* 2010;105(8):1788.
4. Ohman L, Simren M. Pathogenesis of IBS: role of inflammation, immunity and neuroimmune interactions. *Nat Rev Gastroenterol Hepatol.* 2010;7:163-173.
5. Halvorson HA, Schlett CD, Riddle MS. Postinfectious irritable bowel syndrome—a meta-analysis. *Am J Gastroenterol.* 2006;101:1894-1899.
6. Porter CK, Tribble DR, Aliaga PA, Halvorson HA, Riddle MS. Infectious gastroenteritis and risk of developing inflammatory bowel disease. *Gastroenterology.* 2008;135:781-786.
7. Lembo AJ, Neri B, Tolley J, Barken D, Carroll S, Pan H. Use of serum biomarkers in a diagnostic test for irritable bowel syndrome. *Aliment Pharmacol Ther.* 2009;29:834-842.
8. Bercik P, Verdu EF, Collins SM. Is irritable bowel syndrome a low-grade inflammatory bowel disease? *Gastroenterol Clin North Am.* 2005;34:235-245, vi-vii.
9. MacDermott RP. Treatment of irritable bowel syndrome in outpatients with inflammatory bowel disease using a food and beverage intolerance, food and beverage avoidance diet. *Inflamm Bowel Dis.* 2007;13:91-96.

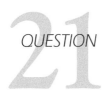

WHAT IS THE ROLE OF BACTERIAL OVERGROWTH IN IBS PATIENTS?

Mark Pimentel, MD

Irritable bowel syndrome (IBS) is a chronic condition that is diagnosed using a characteristic group of symptoms. The symptoms that define IBS include abdominal pain, bloating, and an altered pattern of bowel habits (constipation, diarrhea, or both). Although this condition is one of the most common disorders seen in clinical practice, the cause of these symptoms remains unknown.

A great deal of research has focused on the role of stress and serotonin in the generation of IBS symptoms. Interestingly, however, the symptom of bloating has been largely ignored in clinical trials, despite the fact that bloating is the second most bothersome symptom voiced by IBS patients (abdominal pain is the first). There are many potential explanations why IBS patients have sensations of gas and bloating (eg, visceral hypersensitivity). However, excessive bacterial fermentation may be an important factor.

Recent evidence has emerged to suggest that a proportion of IBS patients suffer from changes in gut ecology. These changes in the gut flora (also referred to as the gut microbiota) can occur for a number of different reasons including postinfectious IBS, altered stool flora due to prior antibiotic use or dietary changes, and small intestinal bacterial overgrowth (SIBO). While data suggest that IBS can begin after a case of acute gastroenteritis (postinfectious IBS), this does not easily explain the persistent symptoms that plague patients, because the original infectious agent (ie, *Campylobacter jejuni, E. coli, Salmonella*, and others) is no longer detectable in the stool. A recent explanation for these ongoing symptoms has become a new "bacterial hypothesis" of IBS. This is believed to be SIBO.

SIBO is a condition defined as excessive bacteria in the small intestine. In most cases, this excessive bacteria arises from the colon (eg, coliform bacteria).[1] In early studies examining subjects with IBS, up to 84% of subjects had SIBO as demonstrated by lactulose breath test.[2] While there are concerns about breath testing as a means of diagnosing SIBO, a recent culture study has shown that some IBS patients indeed have excessive coliform bacteria compared to healthy controls.

Thus, in many patients with IBS, there are excessive numbers of small bowel bacteria, and this can lead to symptoms of gas, bloating, distention, and altered bowel habits. This finding has led to a number of studies that have examined the role of antibiotics in the treatment of IBS. To date there are now six randomized controlled trials demonstrating that antibiotics are effective in improving symptoms of IBS. The most significant of these studies are two phase III multicenter trials of rifaximin in IBS.[3] Rifaximin is a nonabsorbed oral antibiotic that has a high efficacy for treating SIBO, and in these two large-scale studies, this antibiotic demonstrated a significant improvement in IBS after only 14 days of therapy. What is most impressive from the antibiotic studies is that the effect of antibiotics is durable. After 10 to 14 days of antibiotic treatment, IBS subjects remain well for up to 10 weeks. This has never been reported with other drugs in IBS. Previous drug studies in IBS demonstrated benefit while patients were on the drug but immediate relapse with discontinuation of the medication. In the case of rifaximin, subjects noted improvement in their symptoms of bloating for 10 weeks after taking the medication, and this implies that a cause of IBS symptoms has being remedied.

As discussed in other chapters (see Chapters 4 and 5), IBS presents in a number of different ways. Some subjects describe diarrhea while others have symptoms of constipation. It is possible that the gut bacteria may play a role in IBS patients' bowel habits. During the studies of IBS patients that involved breath testing, methane-producing bacteria appeared to be associated with constipation. As well, physiologic studies have demonstrated that methane gas can delay intestinal transit. In a follow-up study, the elimination of methane-producing bacteria with dual antibiotic therapy (rifaximin and neomycin) significantly improved symptoms in IBS patients, especially those with symptoms of constipation.

Overall, I believe that these data suggest that SIBO plays a role in the development and expression of IBS symptoms.[4] What remains to be determined is the cause for SIBO to develop in IBS patients. In most IBS patients, conventional causes of SIBO appear to be absent (eg, prior surgery to the small intestine or colon, small bowel diverticula). Research has thus focused on abnormalities in small bowel motility. It is possible that these abnormalities lead to SIBO, and future treatment may someday lead to the prevention of IBS based on preventing the development of SIBO in IBS patients.

Summary

A large number of studies now demonstrate that in the pathophysiology of IBS, bacteria play a role in symptom generation, confirming a "bacterial hypothesis." Based on breath testing and, more importantly, small bowel culture, this bacterial alteration may be SIBO. While SIBO is not likely to explain symptom expression in all IBS patients,[5] evidence suggests that it may be present in the majority. By identifying a bacterial issue in IBS, antibiotics appear to have beneficial effects on symptoms including bloating, diarrhea, constipation, and abdominal pain. Phase III studies now demonstrate the efficacy of a nonabsorbable antibiotic in nonconstipation IBS (see Chapter 37). In the future, antibiotic treatment will need to be tailored based on the presence or absence of methane compared to hydrogen on breath testing.

References

1. Khoshini R, Dai SC, Lezcano S, et al. A systematic review of diagnostic tests for small intestinal bacterial overgrowth. *Dig Dis Sci.* 2008;53:1443-1454.
2. Pimentel M. Evaluating a "bacterial hypothesis" in IBS using a modification of Koch's postulates. *Am J Gastroenterol.* 2010;105:718-721.
3. Pimentel M, Lembo A, Chey WD, et al. Rifaximin therapy for patients with irritable bowel syndrome without constipation. *N Engl J Med.* 2011;364:22-32.
4. Pimentel M, Lezcano S. Irritable bowel syndrome: bacterial overgrowth—What's known and what to do. *Curr Treat Options Gastroenterol.* 2007;10(4):328-337.
5. Posserud I, Stotzer P-O, Björnsson ES, et al. Small intestinal bacterial overgrowth in patients with irritable bowel syndrome. *Gut.* 2007;56:802-808.

SECTION IV

THE ASSOCIATION OF IBS WITH OTHER MEDICAL CONDITIONS

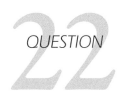
How Common Is Celiac Disease in Patients With IBS?

Joseph Y. Chang, MD, MPH and Yuri A. Saito-Loftus, MD, MPH

Irritable bowel syndrome (IBS) is a common functional gastrointestinal (GI) disorder that is estimated to affect 15% of the population and is characterized by abdominal pain/discomfort with a concurrent disturbance in defecation. In contrast to IBS, celiac disease (CD) is an autoimmune inflammatory enteropathy of the small intestine caused by intolerance to gluten with a prevalence of approximately 1% in the community. Unlike IBS, untreated CD can result in morphologic changes in the small intestinal mucosa that may lead to villous atrophy and malabsorption, and CD patients have higher mortality and malignancy risks compared to the general population. However, similar to IBS patients, patients with CD often present with symptoms of abdominal pain and diarrhea (Table 22-1). Given the similarities in presenting symptoms but dramatically differing outcomes, one may naturally wonder if any patient with suspected IBS should be tested for celiac disease. Testing often seems reasonable, especially in light of reports that as many as 37% of those with CD have an initial diagnosis of IBS.[1] Internists, family physicians, and gastroenterologists are not alone in their struggle with this question as practice guidelines and recommendations from various gastroenterological societies offer differing opinions. Systematic reviews have suggested that serologic testing for CD in patients with IBS may be useful but recommended that further evidence is needed to validate studies indicating an increased prevalence of CD in this population.[2] Furthermore, a cost-effectiveness analysis found that testing for CD was acceptable in patients with IBS but only if the prevalence was above 1%.[3] However, it is unclear whether these recommendations are applicable for all populations given the vastly differing prevalences of both diseases worldwide (Figure 22-1), although in general IBS does appear more prevalent than CD. Therefore, a key clinical and epidemiological question for IBS is, "How common is celiac disease in patients with IBS?"

The answer to this clinical quandary is not as readily apparent as conflicting reports are common. Multiple factors appear to impact findings, and these include the method of

Table 22-1

Comparison of Common Presenting Symptoms of Irritable Bowel Syndrome and Celiac Sprue

Irritable Bowel Syndrome*		Celiac Sprue#	
Presenting Symptom	*%*	*Presenting Symptom*	*%*
Abdominal pain relieved with defecation	69	Diarrhea	54
Abdominal pain not relieved with defecation	31	Weight loss	44
Diarrhea	58	Anemia	35
Constipation	48	Abdominal pain	34
Mucus with bowel movements	32	Bloating	30
Alternating bowel habits—constipation/diarrhea	27	Steatorrhea	26

*Jones R, Lydeard SL. Irritable bowel syndrome in the general population. *BMJ.* 1992;304:87-90.

#Murray JA, Van Dyke C, Plevak MF, et al. Trends in the identification and clinical features of celiac disease in a North American community, 1950-2001. *Clin Gastroenterol Hepatol.* 2003;1:19-27.

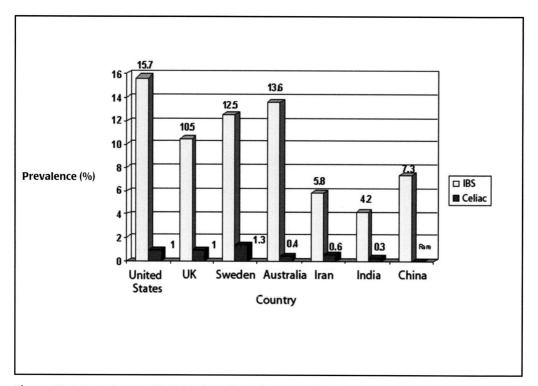

Figure 22-1. Prevalence of irritable bowel syndrome and celiac sprue by country.

diagnosis for CD, the type of serological testing used, and the patient population being investigated. Attempts to better frame this clinical question in terms of type of population investigated is a reasonable approach to this discussion and includes patients with IBS in the community, primary-care setting, secondary care with a gastroenterologist, or referral to a tertiary-care center.

Population-based investigation of IBS is crucial as many patients with IBS do not seek care for their symptoms and those who do seek care may have more severe symptoms and reduced health-related quality of life. From our experience here in Olmsted County, Minnesota, there does not appear to be an increase in prevalence of CD among subjects with IBS in the community. In 2004, Locke and colleagues reported findings from a population-based, case-control study from Olmsted County that included 50 subjects with IBS and 78 asymptomatic healthy controls.[4] CD testing was performed with antiendomysial and tissue transglutaminase (TTg) antibodies in all subjects. The number of subjects who were seropositive for TTg was 2 of 50 (4%) with IBS (95% CI, 0.5% to 13.7%), 2 of 78 (2.6%) in asymptomatic controls (95% CI, 0.3% to 9.0%) ($P=0.64$ IBS versus controls), and the overall prevalence of positive TTg serology was 4%. Although a potential limitation of this study was a type II statistical error given the relatively small sample size, a strength of the study was the comparison with a matched control group from the community. Similar population-based findings were also reported in a study from Sweden that reported no difference in abnormal gluten antibody tests in symptom-free and IBS subjects from a population sample.[5] This was a population-based study from the municipality of Osthammar, Sweden, with a primary aim of evaluating the accuracy of IgA- and IgG-gluten antibodies and endomysium antibodies as screening tools for the diagnosis of CD compared to endoscopy with small bowel biopsies for the histologic diagnosis of CD. A random sample of 50 asymptomatic controls, 50 subjects with dyspepsia, and 50 subjects with IBS were compared. The overall prevalence of an abnormal gluten antibody test was not significantly higher among those with symptoms (24%) than among those who were asymptomatic (20%). Only one subject had a positive antiendomysial antibody test. Therefore, based on the Olmsted County and Swedish experiences, from a population-based approach, it does not appear that undiagnosed CD readily accounts for a significant portion of IBS.

In contrast to the above findings, several studies have reported a higher prevalence of CD in IBS from primary-care, secondary-care, and tertiary-care settings. One such study was the heavily cited report by Sanders and colleagues in the United Kingdom.[6] This case-control study investigated possible celiac disease in 300 patients with IBS (Rome II criteria) and 300 age- and gender-matched healthy controls referred for secondary care at a university hospital. Celiac disease testing was accomplished by measuring serum concentrations of IgG antigliadin, IgA antigliadin, and endomysial antibodies. Not only was a positive association between celiac disease and a diagnosis of IBS found, but also a surprisingly high degree of association between these two disorders. More than 20% of IBS patients had positive antibody test results, and when compared with matched controls, celiac disease and IBS were significantly associated with an odds ratio of 7.0 (95% CI 1.7- to 28.0, $P=0.0004$). This degree of association was impressive and led many to question whether overlooked celiac disease may account for a significant portion of those with IBS symptoms. Similar findings have been reported by the same group from a primary-care based setting with a reported prevalence of CD of 3.3% in subjects with IBS versus 1% from the primary-care population.[7] However, similar findings have not been reported in other populations.

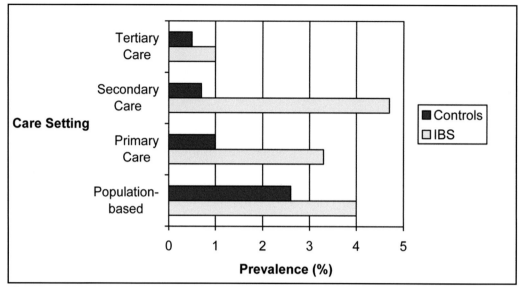

Figure 22-2. Prevalence of celiac disease in irritable bowel syndrome by care setting.

In a secondary care-based study from the Netherlands, 148 patients with IBS were screened for CD by measuring IgA antiendomysial antibodies; total IgA was also measured, and none of the subjects had IgA deficiency.[8] The prevalence of celiac disease in patients presenting with symptoms of IBS was low with none of the IBS subjects found to have elevated endomysial antibodies. Furthermore, 32 of these subjects underwent upper endoscopy with small bowel biopsies, and none had convincing histologic findings for CD. The experience at our large Midwest tertiary medical center also indicates no difference in the prevalence of CD in patients with and without IBS. In yet unpublished data from an ongoing family case-control study of outpatients with and without IBS, of 566 case- and 555 control-probands, 7 cases and 5 controls had a positive or weakly positive TTg test, and 1% of cases and 0.5% of controls were confirmed to have CD by endomysial antibody testing. Therefore, the prevalence of CD in IBS in any type of care setting is uncertain as there appears to be conflicting reports as to whether CD occurs more frequently in IBS (Figure 22-2).

So who do we believe? Do we simply pick a side and say that either celiac disease is common or not common in patients with IBS? Is it even possible to answer this question given that the literature is full of case series or case-control studies that give conflicting results?

A recent well-performed review and meta-analysis on this question by Ford and colleagues has helped to bring some clarity to this question.[9] This analysis involved 14 studies that included 4204 subjects, of whom 2278 (54%) met diagnostic criteria for IBS based on the Manning criteria; Rome I, II, or III; or the Kruis scoring system. It was reported that the pooled prevalence of positive IgA-class antigliadin antibodies, either positive endomysial or TTg antibodies, and biopsy-proved celiac disease was 4.0% (95% CI 1.7 to 7.2), 1.63% (95% CI 0.7 to 3.0), and 4.1% (95% CI 1.9 to 7.0), respectively, with pooled odds ratios of 3.40 (95% CI 1.62-7.13), 2.94 (95% CI 1.36 to 6.35), and 4.34 (95% CI 1.78 to 10.6), respectively. This led to the conclusion that the prevalence of biopsy-proved celiac disease in patients with IBS was approximately 4% and was more than fourfold higher than that of controls without symptoms of IBS.

So does the report by Ford and colleagues settle this controversial question? Unfortunately not. Certainly, many issues still remain regarding the question of how common celiac disease truly is in IBS patients. Factors such as underdiagnosis of celiac disease due to variant forms (eg, latent and atypical), differing diagnostic criteria available for IBS (Manning, Kruis, Rome I, II, or III), and the effect of IgA deficiency on serologic test results all contribute to the difficulties in providing a definitive answer to this clinical question. The impact of ethnicity and gender on the prevalence of CD in IBS is also unclear as most studies are based upon Caucasian populations. Given that CD appears rare in Asians and African Americans, it is unclear if these findings are applicable to those with IBS in these groups. Furthermore, as both IBS and CD have been reported to be more common in women, uncertainty remains if these findings are relevant in men. Complicating this issue further is the identification of a subgroup of patients with IBS with HLA-DQ2 expression and increased CD-associated antibodies that may benefit from a gluten-free diet.[10] Despite these complexities surrounding this clinical question, at this time, it would appear that celiac disease is more common in patients with IBS than the general population. Recent data would indicate a prevalence of celiac disease of 4% in those with IBS versus 1% in the general population.

References

1. Zipser RD, Patel S, Yahya KZ, et al. Presentations of adult celiac disease in a nationwide patient support group. *Dig Dis Sci.* 2003;48:761-764.
2. Cash BD, Schoenfeld P, Chey WD. The utility of diagnostic tests in irritable bowel syndrome patients: a systematic review. *Am J Gastroenterol.* 2002;97:2812-2819.
3. Spiegel BM, DeRosa VP, Gralnek IM, et al. Testing for celiac sprue in irritable bowel syndrome with predominant diarrhea: a cost-effectiveness analysis. *Gastroenterology.* 2004;126:1721-1732.
4. Locke GR, Murray JA, Zinsmeister AR, et al. Celiac disease serology in irritable bowel syndrome and dyspepsia: a population-based case-control study. *Mayo Clin Proc.* 2004;79:476-482.
5. Agreus L, Svardsudd K, Tibblin G, et al. Endomysium antibodies are superior to gliadin antibodies in screening for coeliac disease in patients presenting supposed functional gastrointestinal symptoms. *Scand J Prim Health Care.* 2000;18:105-110.
6. Sanders DS, Carter MJ, Hurlstone DP, et al. Association of adult coeliac disease with irritable bowel syndrome: a case-control study in patients fulfilling ROME II criteria referred to secondary care. *Lancet.* 2001;358: 1504-1508.
7. Sanders DS, Patel D, Stephenson TJ, et al. A primary care cross-sectional study of undiagnosed adult coeliac disease. *Eur J Gastroenterol Hepatol.* 2003;15:407-413.
8. van der Wouden EJ, Nelis GF, Vecht J. Screening for coeliac disease in patients fulfilling the Rome II criteria for irritable bowel syndrome in a secondary care hospital in the Netherlands: a prospective observational study. *Gut.* 2006;444-445.
9. Ford AC, Chey WD, Talley NJ, et al. Yield of diagnostic tests for celiac disease in individuals with symptoms suggestive of irritable bowel syndrome. *Arch Intern Med.* 2009;169:651-658.
10. Wahnschaffe U, Ullrich R, Riecken EO, et al. Celiac disease-like abnormalities in a subgroup of patients with irritable bowel syndrome. *Gastroenterology.* 2001;121:1329-1338.

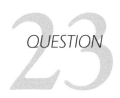
FUNCTIONAL DYSPEPSIA AND IBS: ONE DISEASE OR TWO?

Brian E. Lacy, MD, PhD

Dyspepsia is a highly prevalent disorder that affects up to 25% of the general population. Dyspepsia affects men and women equally and occurs independently of race, religion, and socioeconomic status. Symptoms of dyspepsia include epigastric pain and/or discomfort, early satiety, postprandial fullness, bloating, and nausea. Dyspeptic symptoms may develop due to an organic process (peptic ulcer disease, gastritis, occult acid reflux); however, most patients with dyspeptic symptoms are ultimately diagnosed as having functional dyspepsia (FD).[1] Functional dyspepsia is diagnosed after an appropriate diagnostic evaluation fails to identify an organic etiology to explain the patient's symptoms. Similar to IBS, FD is a chronic disease for many patients, as approximately 50% of patients remain symptomatic over a 5-year follow-up period.[2] Contrary to many patients' beliefs, however, FD is not a risk factor for gastric cancer or peptic ulcer disease.

In an effort to incorporate new information about symptom expression and pathophysiology, the Rome criteria were recently revised (Rome III). Functional dyspepsia is now defined as the presence of symptoms thought to originate in the gastroduodenal region in the absence of any organic, systemic, or metabolic disease likely to explain the symptoms.[3] The Rome committee also introduced two new subcategories to help further differentiate the FD population—postprandial distress syndrome (PDS) and epigastric pain syndrome (EPS; Table 23-1).

Epigastric pain or discomfort is a hallmark symptom in patients with FD. The word discomfort is important to emphasize, as many patients will not complain of pain, but rather state that they have a burning feeling, or pressure, or fullness in the epigastric area. Other common symptoms include early satiety, postprandial fullness and nausea, belching, bloating, and nausea. Frustratingly, symptoms of FD do not consistently predict underlying pathophysiology and do not reliably guide therapy.

The precise etiology of FD is unknown; although there are limited data to suggest that genetics, a prior infection, and environmental factors all play a role in symptom expression. Preliminary studies have demonstrated that patients with the GNβ3 CC genotype are more likely to suffer from dyspepsia. This gene is involved in cell signaling, although

Table 23-1

Rome III Criteria for Functional Dyspepsia

Patients must have one or more of the following symptoms for the past 3 months with symptom onset at least 6 months prior to diagnosis:

- Postprandial fullness
- Early satiety
- Epigastric burning

No evidence of structural disease that is likely to explain symptoms (including upper endoscopy)

Postprandial Distress Syndrome

Diagnostic criteria must include the following:

- Bothersome postprandial fullness, occurring after ordinary-sized meals, at least several times per week
- Early satiation that prevents finishing a regular meal, at least several times per week
- Other symptoms may include the following:
  - Upper abdominal bloating or postprandial nausea or excessive belching
  - Epigastric pain syndrome may coexist

Epigastric Pain Syndrome

Diagnostic criteria must include all of the following:

- Pain or burning localized to the epigastrium, of at least moderate severity at least once per week
- The pain is intermittent
- Not generalized or localized to other abdominal or chest regions
- Not relieved by defecation or passage of flatus
- Not fulfilling criteria for biliary pain
- Other symptoms may include the following:
  - Epigastric pain of a burning quality, but without a retrosternal component
  - Pain induced or relieved by ingestion of a meal, but which also may occur while fasting
- Postprandial distress syndrome may coexist

Modified from Tack J, Talley NJ, Camilleri M, et al. Functional gastroduodenal disorders. *Gastroenterology.* 2006;130:1466-1479.

the exact mechanisms by which alterations in this gene can produce symptoms of dyspepsia are not known. Similar to data from IBS studies, there is evidence demonstrating that a prior gastrointestinal infection may be the cause of FD symptoms in up to 20% of cases. Although *H. pylori* infection may produce dyspeptic symptoms in a small subset of patients, there are few data to support this pathogen as a cause of symptoms in a majority of FD patients. Finally, psychological factors (stress, anxiety, somatization, depression) may modulate symptom expression in some FD patients.

Functional dyspepsia is a heterogeneous disorder, and no single pathophysiologic abnormality can explain the multiple symptoms expressed by FD patients. Research over the past 2 decades has identified a number of different pathophysiologic processes that may disturb normal gastric motor and sensory function in the upper gastrointestinal

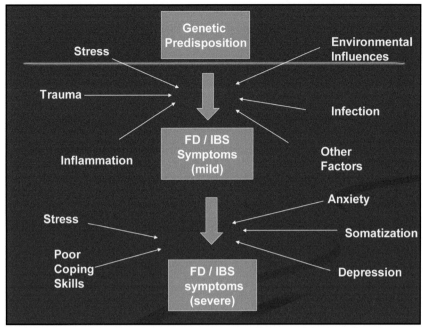

Figure 23-1. Proposed pathway for the development of FD and IBS.

tract of FD patients. Abnormal gastric accommodation may account for symptoms of epi gastric fullness and pressure in some patients and is present in approximately 40% of FD patients.[1] Antral hypomotility and delayed gastric emptying are present in other patients with FD, with several studies showing that approximately one-third of FD patients have a mild delay in gastric emptying. Similar to many IBS patients, FD patients are character-ized by visceral hypersensitivity. Balloon distension studies have demonstrated that up to two-thirds of patients with FD have heightened gastric perception, although this does not correlate with any specific symptom. Other patients with FD may have gastric electrical dysrhythmias, abnormalities of duodenal motor or sensory function, or disordered feed-back from the proximal small intestine as the cause of their symptoms.

Why Might FD and IBS Overlap?

There are several plausible theories to explain why FD and IBS might overlap. One, they are both common medical disorders. The prevalence of IBS is 12% to 15% in the United States, while the prevalence of FD is approximately 10%. Given the high prevalence of both disorders, it would not be uncommon for some patients to suffer from both disor-ders. Two, the proposed etiologies of FD seem remarkably similar to those of IBS (see Chapter 13). A number of research studies have shown that, for both conditions, a genetic predisposition may exist (Figure 23-1). For FD symptoms to develop, however, the GI tract must be exposed or subjected to some type of insult. This may be the result of a viral or bacterial infection (ie, postinfectious FD), an inflammatory process (ie, medications), or stress (eg, mental, physical, emotional, financial, sexual). Symptoms of IBS and/or FD may then develop, and these are generally mild. However, symptoms may become severe if psychological factors are present and burdensome (ie, anxiety, depression, somatization, catastrophization, poor coping skills, ongoing stress). Three, both FD and IBS are linked by similar pathophysiology. As mentioned above, two-thirds of patients with FD have evidence of visceral hypersensitivity, demonstrated during balloon distention studies. Thus, it is easy to think of FD as nothing more than IBS pathophysiology expressed in the upper gastrointestinal tract. Finally, IBS and FD are similar in that they both respond, in part, to treatments for visceral hypersensitivity and visceral pain[4] (see below).

What Treatment Options Are Available for My Patient With FD?

DIET

Most patients with FD have symptoms associated with the ingestion of food.[5] There are limited data to suggest that dietary fat may increase gastric sensitivity to distension and cause dyspeptic symptoms. I recommend that patients with FD focus on low-fat meals and smaller, more frequent meals.

ERADICATION OF *H. PYLORI*

Testing and treating for *H. pylori* (if present) is often recommended as the first step in the management of younger patients with uncomplicated dyspeptic symptoms. Although safe, this strategy is unlikely to improve symptoms of FD. In fact, a recent analysis found only a small benefit above placebo, with a number needed to treat of 14.

ANTISECRETORY THERAPY

Histamine-receptor-type-2-antagonists (H2RAs) are marginally better than placebo at improving epigastric pain, although they do not improve other dyspeptic symptoms. Most providers thus use a proton pump inhibitor (PPI) as first-line treatment for FD. This is not an unreasonable course of action, as short-term risks of PPIs are low, and this may provide relief of symptoms in a small number of people, many of whom may have had silent acid reflux. Overall, however, PPIs are only approximately 10% better than placebo at improving dyspeptic symptoms with a number needed to treat (NNT) of 9. In addition, long-term use of PPIs can be expensive, and there are emerging data that long-term PPI use may place patients at increased risk for *Clostridium difficile* colitis, community-acquired pneumonia, and hip fractures.

PROKINETIC AGENTS

FD patients with symptoms of early satiety, epigastric fullness, and postprandial discomfort may respond to the use of prokinetic agents. Metoclopramide and domperidone are now the most commonly employed agents. Although individual patients may respond to prokinetic medications, there are conflicting data in the literature regarding their utility, with one systematic review showing prokinetic agents were somewhat better than placebo, while a meta-analysis did not show any benefits compared to placebo. In addition, metoclopramide is associated with a variety of side effects (anxiety, drowsiness, decreased libido, breast tenderness) and as of February 2009 carries a black-box warning. Domperidone is not readily available in the US and is difficult to obtain for most providers.

ANTIDEPRESSANTS

Tricyclic antidepressants (TCAs) may improve symptoms of dyspepsia in patients who have failed H2RAs, PPIs, or prokinetic agents. Although the precise mechanism is unknown, they may improve symptoms of visceral hypersensitivity and reduce intragastric pressure. In general, lower doses of TCAs are used to treat FD than depression. Selective serotonin reuptake inhibitors (SSRIs) have not been well-studied for the treatment of FD, although a recent trial of venlafaxine failed to show any benefits over placebo.

HYPNOTHERAPY AND PSYCHOLOGICAL THERAPIES

Hypnotherapy may improve dyspeptic symptoms in some patients, and a recent study found that hypnotherapy was better than medical therapy and supportive therapy at improving quality of life and symptom scores (see Chapter 45). Although not well studied, psychological therapies, including cognitive behavioral therapy, may relieve symptoms of dyspepsia by reducing coexisting stress and anxiety (see Chapter 46).

Summary

Managing patients with IBS and FD can be a challenging and frustrating process for clinicians. Currently, these two common functional gastrointestinal disorders are thought of as completely separate disorders. Because many patients have overlapping symptoms of IBS and dyspepsia, maintaining two separate diagnoses leads to separate, but often parallel, processes of evaluation and treatment. Unfortunately, this results in redundant laboratory tests, duplication of diagnostic studies, frequent office visits, and the use of multiple medications.

As discussed, IBS and FD are remarkably similar. Injury to the enteric nervous system likely serves as the unifying link in the generation and expression of the typical symptoms found in IBS and FD. Some patients will manifest the abnormal pathophysiology that develops as a result of ENS injury with primarily upper GI tract symptoms (epigastric fullness and discomfort, bloating, nausea), while others will manifest primarily lower GI symptoms (abdominal pain and disordered defecation).

The recognition that symptom expression in IBS and FD reflects different manifestations of the same disorder should help eliminate repetitive diagnostic testing, minimize office visits, and improve our ability to target therapy at the common link. Treatment options for IBS and FD should be directed at modulating both peripheral and central pain mechanisms, with the goal of improving symptoms, improving quality of life, and minimizing the economic burden to society.[6]

References

1. Tack J, Caenepeel, P, Fischler B, et al. Symptoms associated with hypersensitivity to gastric distention in functional dyspepsia. *Gastroenterology.* 2001;121:526-535.
2. Talley NJ, Dennis EH, Schettler-Duncan VA, et al. Overlapping upper and lower gastrointestinal symptoms in irritable bowel syndrome patients with constipation or diarrhea. *Am J Gastroenterol.* 2003;98:2454-2459.
3. Tack J, Talley NJ, Camilleri M, et al. Functional gastroduodenal disorders. *Gastroenterology.* 2006;130: 1466-1479.
4. Saad RJ, Chey WD. Review article: current and emerging therapies for functional dyspepsia. *Aliment Pharmacol Ther.* 2006;24:475-492.
5. Bisschops R, Karamanolis G, Arts J, et al. Relationship between symptoms and ingestion of a meal in functional dyspepsia. *Gut.* 2008;57:1495-1503.
6. Lacy BE, Cash BD. Clinical cornerstone. A 32 year old woman with abdominal pain. *JAMA.* 2008;299:555-565.

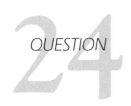
WHAT IS THE RELATIONSHIP BETWEEN GERD AND IBS?

Ronnie Fass, MD, FACP, FACG and Tiberiu Hershcovici, MD

Gastroesophageal reflux disease (GERD) and irritable bowel syndrome (IBS) are 2 disorders commonly found in the general population. The prevalence of IBS in North America ranges from 3% to 20%, with most prevalence estimates ranging from 10% to 15%. GERD is also highly prevalent. Population-based studies demonstrate that 32% to 57% of the general adult population in Western countries had typical GERD-related symptoms within the past year. The community prevalence of weekly heartburn ranges from 10% to 21%. Interestingly, both GERD and IBS are less common in Asia than in Western populations. For example, the reported population prevalence of GERD in East Asia ranges from 3% to 7% for weekly symptoms of heartburn and/or acid regurgitation.

The classic symptoms of GERD are heartburn and acid regurgitation. Extraesophageal and atypical symptoms of GERD may include wheezing, chronic cough, hoarseness, chest pain, belching, and sleep deprivation. However, a variety of other symptoms have been seen in GERD patients. These include flatulence, abdominal discomfort, and alterations in bowel movements.

The symptoms of IBS have been well described (see Chapters 4 through 6). Suffice it to say that the clinical presentation of IBS can be quite diverse. Many IBS patients report a wide range of colonic and extra-colonic symptoms, which may include symptoms referable to the upper gastrointestinal tract, including symptoms of reflux.

Most epidemiological studies show a significant overlap between the different functional disorders of the digestive tract in the general population. Consequently, the presence of IBS-related symptoms in patients with GERD may suggest an overlap between two distinct disorders that share a similar pathophysiologic mechanism, such as visceral hypersensitivity or gastrointestinal (GI) dysmotility. Alternatively, lower abdominal symptoms may be part of the overall clinical presentation of GERD, suggesting that the underlying mechanism for GERD may lead to upper as well as lower gut symptoms.

There are 2 principal hypotheses regarding the relationship between GERD- and IBS-related symptoms.[1] The first theory suggests that GERD and IBS are both highly prevalent disorders and thus statistically are likely to overlap in a significant number of patients. The second theory, which is more controversial, proposes that IBS-like symptoms are part of the spectrum of GERD presentation. Implicit in either theory is that these two disorders may be linked pathophysiologically by altered visceral sensation or disordered gastrointestinal motility. We will now present the data to support these two different hypotheses.

IBS-like symptoms are very common among GERD patients. Depending on the criteria used to diagnose IBS, between 19% and 71% of GERD patients also have IBS. In one population-based study that explored the relationship between IBS, GERD, and bronchial hyper-responsiveness (BHR) using a symptom questionnaire, the 12-month prevalence of IBS-related symptoms for men and women was 10.5% and 22.9%, respectively. The 12-month prevalence of GERD-related symptoms was 29.4% and 28.2%, respectively. Of the 910 subjects who were found to have GERD, 19% reported IBS-like symptoms; of the 546 IBS patients, 32% were found to have GERD. The authors reported that IBS and GERD symptoms occurred more frequently together than expected and that the conditions are independently associated with each other. Another study evaluated GERD patients seeking care and demonstrated that IBS is more prevalent in GERD patients than in the general population (35% versus 0.6% to 6%). In another smaller study, the prevalence of IBS, as defined by Rome I criteria, was determined in subjects with GERD as compared with non-GERD controls. Of the 35 GERD subjects, 71% were positive for IBS, whereas only 35% of the 49 non-GERD control subjects had IBS. The study demonstrated that the prevalence of IBS was significantly more common in the GERD group than in the non-GERD group. Additionally, in this study, a subset of GERD patients underwent 24-hour esophageal pH monitoring, and 64% of those with IBS had abnormal pH test results.

In a recent systematic review of the literature evaluating the prevalence of IBS and GERD in the general population and the rate of overlapping symptoms between both disorders, the average prevalence of GERD was 19.4% while that of IBS was 12.1%.[2] Several of the included studies determined that the GERD maximum mean prevalence in patients already diagnosed with IBS was 39.3%. There was a significant variability in the GERD prevalence, ranging from 17% to 80%. The likely reason for the wide range of GERD prevalence in IBS patients appeared to depend on the method for diagnosing GERD. The maximum mean prevalence of IBS in subjects with already-known GERD was 48.8%. The prevalence of IBS in GERD patients also had a wide range (31% to 71%) and was clearly dependent on the criteria used to diagnose IBS (Manning, Rome I, or Rome II). This systematic review demonstrated that IBS and GERD appear to overlap to a degree that is greater than their individual prevalence in the community. The authors concluded that the prevalence of IBS in the non-GERD community was only 5.1%. These data suggested strong overlap between GERD and IBS and postulated that IBS appears to be relatively uncommon in the absence of GERD.

Several studies examining extra-colonic features of IBS clearly demonstrated that these patients frequently report typical GERD-related symptoms. The relationship between GERD and functional GI disorders has been primarily studied in IBS patients. The prevalence of GERD is higher in IBS patients than in the general population and varies from 11% to 52%.

In another study, the nature and the frequency of gastroesophageal reflux symptoms were assessed in 25 patients with IBS. Symptoms such as heartburn, acid regurgitation, and dysphagia were significantly more common in IBS patients than in an age- and gender-matched control group. Esophageal symptoms were present daily in 28% and once a week in 52% of the IBS patients. Ambulatory 24-hour esophageal pH monitoring showed abnormal esophageal acid exposure in 50% of the IBS patients. This study also demonstrated that significant reduction in lower esophageal sphincter pressure accompanies IBS, but no disturbances of esophageal body motor activity could be found. The results of this study provided clear confirmation that esophageal symptoms are significantly more common in IBS patients than in the general population.

Last, there is a limited amount of data regarding GERD symptoms in IBS patients based on their subtype. One study enrolled consecutive patients with IBS who were classified according to their leading complaint (constipation or diarrhea predominant). Overlap with GERD-related symptoms was observed in 32.9% of the IBS-constipation predominant and 40.9% of the IBS-diarrhea predominant patients.

In contrast to the data presented above showing that GERD is more common in patients with IBS, some studies have shown that heartburn, which is a common complaint in IBS, was reported by nearly one-third of patients but was observed just as frequently as in the control group.

If one accepts the hypothesis that IBS and GERD are closely linked, are there pathophysiologic mechanisms that might be responsible for this close association? Recent studies in twins have suggested that there is probably a distinct genetic contribution to the development of both IBS and GERD. Genetic modeling confirmed the independent additive genetic effects in GERD and IBS, with estimates of genetic variance of 22% in IBS and 13% in GERD. Alternatively, some authors have postulated that IBS patients may have motility disturbances similar to those seen in GERD in the upper GI tract. Ineffective esophageal motility and impaired primary peristalsis have been suggested to be contributing factors to the pathophysiology of GERD. In IBS, alteration in colonic transit and small bowel motility are demonstrable in some patients. Thus, some authors have speculated that generalized smooth-muscle dysfunction of the GI tract may explain the close relationship between IBS and GERD. As noted previously, one small study evaluating esophageal function in IBS subjects demonstrated a significant reduction in lower esophageal sphincter basal pressure. These findings could explain GERD-related symptoms in IBS patients.

Several other studies have suggested that GERD and IBS overlap because of general visceral hyperalgesia. Visceral hyperalgesia, particularly rectal hyperalgesia, has long been associated with IBS. It has been shown that IBS subjects have lower rectal sensory thresholds for pain as compared to healthy controls and concomitantly exhibited significantly lower sensory thresholds for both perception and discomfort in the esophagus.[3] Furthermore, investigators have also demonstrated that IBS subjects have a significantly lower threshold for esophageal symptoms during esophageal provocative testing (Bethanechol subcutaneously and the balloon distension test), but there was no difference in esophageal motility or lower esophageal sphincter basal pressure when compared with controls. The authors hypothesized that IBS subjects do not have pathologic reflux but are rather more sensitive to physiologic reflux. In support of this concept, GERD patients who also had IBS perceived their symptoms as more severe and tended not to achieve the same degree of improvement in GERD symptoms when treated with a

PPI as those without IBS. Other studies have shown that bowel symptoms were associated with reflux symptom scores but not with esophageal acid exposure, again supporting the importance of visceral hypersensitivity in these patients.

The influence of IBS and psychological distress on the response to proton pump inhibitor (PPI) therapy in patients with GERD has been recently evaluated.[4] Patients with IBS reported more severe GERD symptoms at baseline but experienced a similar magnitude of improvement in GERD symptoms as compared to patients without IBS while on PPI therapy. The authors found that comorbid IBS and psychological distress, but not the presence or absence of erosive esophagitis, influenced symptom perception and disease-specific quality of life before and after PPI therapy.

The second theory to explain the relationship between GERD and IBS is that IBS symptoms are part of the typical GERD presentation. Some studies suggest that IBS-like symptoms represent an extra-esophageal, but GI-related, manifestation of GERD. Evidence to support this hypothesis originates from therapeutic trials in GERD patients. In these studies, lower abdominal symptoms, suggestive of IBS, significantly improved after medical or surgical anti-reflux treatment. In one study, up to 24% of patients with GERD reported a significant or complete improvement of their bowel symptoms following acid suppressive therapy, mainly using PPIs. In another study, 30% of GERD patients who underwent laparoscopic fundoplication were found to have IBS using Rome II criteria, and, of these patients, 81% reported significant improvement in their IBS symptoms postoperatively.

In another study, investigators reported that 41% of patients with GERD and IBS reported complete resolution of their IBS symptoms after receiving esomeprazole 20 mg daily for 3 months. However, the results of this study should be interpreted cautiously because of the lack of a placebo arm.

The underlying pathophysiological mechanism that explains how gastroesophageal reflux can cause IBS-like symptoms has yet to be elucidated. It is likely that the recently growing interest in the full spectrum of GERD symptoms, which includes atypical and extra-esophageal manifestations as well as sleep abnormalities, has led to the recognition that lower abdominal complaints may also be encountered in patients with GERD.

Additional support for the concept that GERD is a more systemic disorder than is currently accepted was provided by the recently introduced GERD questionnaire, the ReQuest (Nycomed; Constance, Germany). The developers of the ReQuest incorporated lower GI complaints suggestive of IBS into the questionnaire after demonstrating that patients and physicians perceive that these symptoms are part of the symptom spectrum of GERD. Therapeutic studies that used the ReQuest as an evaluative tool clearly demonstrated a significant reduction in lower abdomen and dyspepsia-like symptoms in response to PPI therapy.

Summary

Several studies clearly demonstrate that GERD is highly prevalent in IBS patients and vice versa. The reason for this close relationship between the two disorders remains unknown. Presently, there are two leading hypotheses that attempt to explain this relationship. The first suggests that IBS-like symptoms are part of the spectrum of GERD manifestations. The other suggests that IBS and GERD are two different disorders that are both highly prevalent with a similar underlying pathophysiology. Both hypotheses need to be further evaluated.

References

1. Gasiorowska A, Poh CH, Fass R. Gastroesophageal reflux disease (GERD) and irritable bowel syndrome (IBS)—Is it one disease or an overlap of two disorders? *Dig Dis Sci.* 2009;54:1829-1834.
2. Nastaskin I, Mehdikhani Conklin J, Park S, Pimentel M. Studying the overlap between IBS and GERD: a systematic review of the literature. *Dig Dis Sci.* 2006;51:2113-2120.
3. Trimble KC, Farouk R, Pryde A, Douglas S, Heading RC. Heightened visceral sensation in functional gastrointestinal disease is not site-specific. Evidence for a generalized disorder of gut sensitivity. *Dig Dis Sci.* 1995;40:1607-1613.
4. Nojkov B, Rubenstein JH, Adlis SA, et al. The influence of co-morbid IBS and psychological distress on outcomes and quality of life following PPI therapy in patients with gastro-oesophageal reflux disease. *Aliment Pharmacol Ther.* 2008;27:473-482.

WHAT OTHER COMMON GI DISORDERS OCCUR IN PATIENTS WITH IBS?

Max J. Schmulson, MD

Patients with irritable bowel syndrome (IBS) commonly have a variety of gastrointestinal and extraintestinal manifestations. A twofold increase in these comorbidities has been reported. Gastrointestinal manifestations include gastroesophageal reflux, dyspepsia, functional constipation, fecal incontinence, and lactose intolerance. More recently, there has been increased attention paid to a possible relationship with disorders such as celiac disease and inflammatory bowel disease (Figure 25-1). In this chapter, I will address these common comorbid gastrointestinal disorders.

Gastroesophageal Reflux Disease (GERD)

GERD is present in up to 39% of patients with IBS, and IBS has been shown to be an independent risk factor for GERD.[1] We have found that heartburn is present in up to one-half of volunteers who fulfill criteria for IBS. Heartburn is a highly specific symptom of gastroesophageal reflux, and data from our clinic show that 60% of patients reporting this symptom have acid reflux as demonstrated by pH monitoring.[2] From these findings, we can speculate that approximately two-thirds of IBS patients reporting heartburn will have true acid reflux and one-third will have functional heartburn. There are reports that suggest that a common link between IBS and GERD exists; however, there is no convincing evidence for a common underlying pathophysiology, such as visceral hypersensitivity, a motility abnormality, or somatization (see Chapter 24).[3]

As for the approach to these patients, unless there are alarm symptoms such as dysphagia, bleeding, anemia, or weight loss, I recommend treating them as usual, with a trial of a proton pump inhibitor (PPI) for a period of 8 to 12 weeks and even repeating a treatment period. Whether to use a single dose PPI or double dose is controversial. In the literature, there are more reports of the presence of IBS in patients with GERD than reports of GERD in IBS patients, and these studies have concluded that the presence of IBS is related to worsened GERD symptoms, more treatment failures, psychological

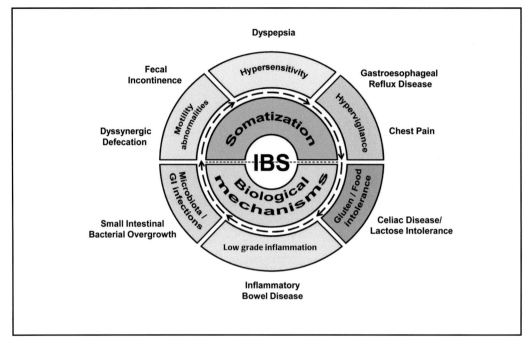

Figure 25-1. The underlying pathophysiological mechanisms for the common gastrointestinal disorders that can occur in IBS are unknown. We can probably classify these comorbid conditions as those related to somatization and those that have a biological mechanism. However, we can hypothesize that even using this classification system, the clinical manifestations may be the consequence of somatization, but, at the same time, may represent expression of a biological mechanism. For example, symptoms of gastroesophageal reflux in IBS may be a manifestation of somatization, but acid-related inflammation of the esophageal mucosa that stimulates sensory nerves can also generate symptoms, such as heartburn. Conversely, celiac disease (gluten malabsorption) can coexist with IBS, but, at the same time, it is possible that a gluten-sensitive mechanism may exacerbate or generate IBS symptoms (eg, bloating and pain), as well. More research is needed to identify the underlying causes of these comorbidities and/or clinical manifestations.

distress, and a negative impact on health-related quality of life. There is evidence that patients with GERD who have extraesophageal manifestations such as IBS may not respond to a standard dose of PPI and may need a higher dose, and one may expect that the presence of GERD in IBS would have the same outcome. Therefore, I always start with a double dose of PPI in patients with IBS and GERD, and if there is no clinical response after two treatment periods, I then study the patient objectively.

We have also found that belching is commonly present in subjects with IBS. It is reported by up to 55% of patients, mainly men with IBS, but it is also very frequent in controls without any functional gastrointestinal disorder. Therefore, its clinical significance, and whether its presence deserves diagnostic evaluation to rule out GERD, needs to be further investigated. Finally, chest pain is another symptom that is very frequent in IBS and can be related to GERD.[2]

Dyspepsia

In a systematic review on comorbidities in IBS, Riedl and colleagues found reports that 40% of IBS patients also have dyspeptic symptoms, such as epigastric pain, or sensations of abdominal fullness, distension, early satiety, and vomiting.[3] We found that epigastric pain and nausea were present in 54% and 21% of volunteers with IBS and were more commonly reported than in controls without IBS (44% and 12%, respectively[2]). Data from our laboratory have also shown that symptoms of early satiety and upper abdominal fullness were more frequent in patients with diarrhea predominant IBS (IBS-D) than in those with constipation (IBS-C).

Dyspepsia is a strong predictor for IBS-related consulting behavior, and it has been suggested that subjects suffering from both disorders consult physicians for similar reasons.[4] Again, it is possible that these comorbidities might arise from common underlying pathophysiologic mechanisms. However, in their systematic review, Riedl and colleagues found that the presence of IBS is independent of functional dyspepsia and other gastrointestinal disorders.[3]

Functional Anorectal Disorders

Irritable bowel syndrome, slow transit constipation, and pelvic floor dysfunction are the three primary symptom-based constipation groups. Each one has a different pathophysiological basis, and pelvic floor dysfunction may be present in up to one half of patients with IBS. Although constipation is one of the IBS subgroups, in patients not responding to treatment or in those with symptoms of obstructive defecation, pelvic floor dyssynergia needs to be ruled out.

In contrast to symptoms of constipation, Whitehead and colleagues reported that fecal incontinence was present in 1.2% of patients with IBS, five times more than the prevalence in controls without IBS or without inflammatory bowel disease.[5] The clinical importance of fecal incontinence in IBS is that it can overwhelm IBS-D patients who already suffer from symptoms of diarrhea and urgency. In addition, incontinence can also occur in patients with IBS and constipation as liquid stool and mucus can leak around hard stool in the rectum. Finally, fecal incontinence has a significant impact on patients' quality of life (see Chapter 27). Patients usually will not bring this embarrassing issue to the attention of their healthcare provider. Thus, we as clinicians should be aware of its presence in IBS patients and raise the issue when appropriate.

Inflammatory Bowel Disease

There has been an interest lately in the possible role of low-grade inflammation in IBS, and some data suggest that IBS may be part of a spectrum of inflammatory bowel disorders (IBD). In addition, symptoms of IBS may be present in IBD patients in remission. Several studies have found a significantly elevated incidence of intestinal comorbidities that have a biomarker-based diagnosis such as IBD, malabsorption, bowel obstruction, and diverticulitis in IBS patients.[5] It has been suggested that these comorbidities may reflect the ambiguity of making a symptom-based diagnosis of IBS in the presence of these organic disorders, which can generate symptoms similar to those of IBS.[5] In my opinion, this may explain the earlier belief that the "irritable colon" might be the initial manifestation of IBD. Hence, it is important to perform a colonoscopy in IBS patients with rectal bleeding, a family history of IBD, and those patients with persistent symptoms, and, of course, for screening purposes, those older than 50 years of age.

Celiac Disease

Celiac disease (CD) may have symptoms similar to those of IBS, including diarrhea, abdominal bloating or distension, and abdominal pain (see Chapter 22). Current guidelines recommend an IBS diagnosis based on symptom criteria, limited diagnostic testing, and consideration for investigating possible CD in IBS patients with diarrhea. A recent cost-effective analysis has determined that IBS-D patients should be tested for CD in countries with a prevalence of CD higher than 1% in the general population.[6] Lately, there has been an increased interest in the relationship between IBS and CD, and, in fact, there has been a hypothesis of a "gluten sensitive" IBS. Ford and colleagues reported a biopsy-proven CD prevalence of 4.1% in IBS, a fourfold increase compared to controls. Interestingly, there was no difference according to the IBS bowel habit predominance, suggesting that CD may be considered not only in those with IBS-D, but also in those with IBS-C or IBS-A.[7]

Small Intestinal Bacterial Overgrowth

The pathogenesis of IBS has been related to abnormalities of the gut microbiota, small intestinal bacterial overgrowth (SIBO), and gastrointestinal infections (postinfectious IBS; see Chapter 18). In a systematic review, Ford and colleagues recently reported that the prevalence of SIBO in subjects with IBS is between 4% and 64% depending on the type of test performed (lactulose or glucose hydrogen breath test, jejunal aspirate, and culture) with a three- to fivefold increase in the odds ratio for a positive test in IBS patients compared to healthy asymptomatic controls.[8] The majority of the studies in this review were from tertiary referral centers; therefore, the data may not be generalizable to patients in primary care or to the general population. On the other hand, there is no currently accepted validated test or gold standard to diagnose SIBO. There is evidence, however, that supports the use of nonabsorbed oral antibiotics for the treatment of IBS symptoms in a subgroup of patients with IBS. Whether SIBO is a pathogenic factor, or whether it plays a role in symptom generation in IBS, remains to be elucidated; however, I do not believe that there is any need to routinely test all patients for SIBO before initiating a treatment plan using a nonabsorbable antibiotic.

Lactose Intolerance

Patients with IBS often report alimentary intolerance and tend to eliminate dairy and other products from their diet. Probably the most commonly reported food intolerance by IBS patients is lactose intolerance. This is closely followed by fructose intolerance, due to the fact that they are both highly fermentable substrates that can contribute to symptoms such as bloating, abdominal distension, or changes in bowel habit. The prevalence of lactose or fructose malabsorption, using hydrogen breath tests, is approximately one-third of all IBS patients, which is similar to the frequency in the general population. Currently, genetic markers for hypolactasia are available as a diagnostic tool for lactose intolerance and can predict its relationship with symptoms in patients with IBS.

References

1. Nastaskin I, Mehdikhani E, Conklin J, Park S, Pimentel M. Studying the overlap between IBS and GERD: a systematic review of the literature. *Dig Dis Sci.* 2006;51:2113-2120.
2. Schmulson M, Pulido D, Escobar C, Farfán-Labone B, Gutiérrez-Reyes G, López-Alvarenga JC. Heartburn and other related symptoms are independent of body mass index in irritable bowel syndrome. *Rev Esp Enferm Dig.* 2010;102:229-233.
3. Riedl A, Schmidtmann M, Stengel A, et al. Somatic comorbidities of irritable bowel syndrome: a systematic analysis. *J Psychosom Res.* 2008;64:573-582.
4. Ford AC, Forman D, Bailey AG, Axon AT, Moayyedi P. Irritable bowel syndrome: a 10-yr natural history of symptoms and factors that influence consultation behavior. *Am J Gastroenterol.* 2008;103:1229-1239.
5. Whitehead WE, Palsson OS, Levy RR, Feld AD, Turner M, Von Korff M. Comorbidity in irritable bowel syndrome. *Am J Gastroenterol.* 2007;102:2767-2776.
6. Spiegel BM, DeRosa VP, Gralnek IM, Wang V, Dulai GS. Testing for celiac sprue in irritable bowel syndrome with predominant diarrhea: a cost-effectiveness analysis. *Gastroenterology.* 2004;126:1721-1732.
7. Ford AC, Chey WD, Talley NJ, Malhotra A, Spiegel BM, Moayyedi P. Yield of diagnostic tests for celiac disease in individuals with symptoms suggestive of irritable bowel syndrome: systematic review and meta-analysis. *Arch Intern Med.* 2009;169:651-658.
8. Ford AC, Spiegel BM, Talley NJ, Moayyedi P. Small intestinal bacterial overgrowth in irritable bowel syndrome: systematic review and meta-analysis. *Clin Gastroenterol Hepatol.* 2009;7:1279-1286.

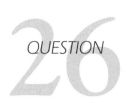
FROM WHICH NONGASTROINTESTINAL DISORDERS ARE PATIENTS WITH IBS MOST LIKELY TO SUFFER?

Susan Lucak, MD and Rupa Mukherjee, MD

Nongastrointestinal disorders have been reported in twice as many patients with irritable bowel syndrome (IBS) as compared to healthy controls. These comorbid disorders reduce IBS patients' quality of life and increase healthcare seeking. The excess healthcare costs associated with the diagnosis of IBS are due mostly to these comorbid conditions. IBS patients not only have an excess number of nongastrointestinal somatic disorders but also an increased number of psychiatric diagnoses. A number of theories have been proposed to explain the association of IBS with nongastrointestinal disorders; however, a single, unifying pathophysiologic mechanism has yet to be identified.

Pathophysiology

IBS is a heterogeneous condition whose exact etiology is unknown, although it is likely multifactorial in nature. It has been suggested that IBS results from a complex interplay of visceral hypersensitivity, autonomic nervous system dysregulation, modification in smooth muscle reactivity, alteration in immune function, and dysregulation in brain processing.

The idea that dysfunction at the level of the central nervous system may be involved in the pathophysiology of IBS is supported by functional brain magnetic resonance imaging (fMRI) studies performed by Naliboff, Chang, and others.[1,2] Their work has shown that patients with IBS process pain by activating regions of the brain different from healthy controls. One seminal study illustrated this finding by investigating the pain response of IBS patients to rectal distension. It was found that IBS patients, unlike healthy controls, activated specific regions of the brain, such as the middle and posterior cingulate gyrus, which are associated with enhanced pain processing, both during and in anticipation of painful rectal distension.[1] The same group also investigated brain responses to visceral and somatic stimuli in patients with IBS with and without fibromyalgia. They found chronic stimulus-specific enhancement of the anterior cingulate cortex in response to sensory stimuli in both syndromes, suggesting a possible pathophysiologic connection in these two chronic pain syndromes.

In 2007, Whitehead and coworkers conducted a study to determine whether IBS patients are at increased risk to develop specific comorbid disorders or whether they simply over-reported their symptoms.[3] They could not identify a unique association between IBS and other nongastrointestinal somatic disorders that might suggest a shared pathophysiology or risk factor. Instead, they reported that IBS comorbidity was due to a general amplification of symptom reporting. Another question they posed was whether IBS somatic comorbidity could be explained by psychiatric disease. Their results show that comorbidity was influenced, but not explained, by psychiatric illness and that it was due to hypervigilance for noticing sensations and to a lower threshold for consulting a physician. Surprisingly, somatic comorbidity in their study was noted only in 16% of IBS patients. Thus, although it seems to make sense that IBS and its associated painful conditions share common pathophysiology, there are likely other factors critical to the generation and expression of pain in these disorders.

Whitehead and others also confirmed that comorbid psychiatric disorders were more prevalent in IBS patients (51.2%).[3] Patients with psychiatric diagnoses had significantly more comorbid somatic diagnoses than IBS patients without psychiatric diagnoses, suggesting that psychological symptoms contribute to excess comorbidity. However, IBS patients without psychiatric comorbidity still had more comorbid somatic diagnoses than controls.

Nongastrointestinal Disorders Associated With Irritable Bowel Syndrome

Nongastrointestinal disorders that are most frequently associated with IBS can be divided into somatic and psychiatric categories.

SOMATIC DISORDERS[3,4]

- **Fibromyalgia**, a chronic condition characterized by diffuse musculoskeletal pain with specific tender points, is a common disorder associated with IBS. This association has been most frequently investigated. A number of studies report an average occurrence of 32.5% (range, 28%-65%) in patients with IBS.

  Specific musculoskeletal conditions that are also associated with IBS are low back pain (38%), tendonitis (30%), arthralgia (26%), and neck pain (17%).

- **Temporomandibular joint disorder (TMJ)** is an orofacial pain syndrome characterized by restricted movement of the jaw and clenching of the jaw. TMJ is reportedly found in 16% of patients with IBS. Catechol-O-methyltransferase (COMT) polymorphism has been associated with pain sensitivity and TMJ. COMT polymorphism has not been investigated in IBS.

- **Chronic headaches** have been reported in up to 50% to 60% of patients with IBS, a prevalence rate significantly higher than healthy subjects. A study conducted in Denmark followed IBS patients who presented with headaches for a period of 5 to 7 years. Those patients whose IBS symptoms improved also reported an improvement in their headaches compared to those whose IBS symptoms persisted, in which case their headaches also tended to persist. These results suggest that somatic comorbidity may be an indicator of a more severe disease course in some IBS patients. Of note, migraine headaches occur in only 6% of IBS patients, a prevalence rate no different than the general population.

- **Chronic fatigue syndrome (CFS)** is seen in approximately 14% of IBS patients as determined by a single study. In the general population, the prevalence of CFS is only 0.4%. Conversely, in CFS patients, the occurrence of IBS ranges from 35% to 92% (median, 51%). There is no evidence for IBS and CFS having similar abnormalities in their immune function. Both conditions are associated with anxiety and depression, which may be a potential link between these two disorders.

- **Sleep disturbances** have been reported in up to 33% of IBS patients compared to 11% of healthy controls. Rapid eye movement (REM) sleep is twice as frequent in IBS patients compared to controls, leading to a less restful sleep. Poor sleep was found to lead to higher rates of gastrointestinal symptoms on the following day in women with IBS.

- **Chronic pelvic pain** is reported in up to 49.9% of female patients suffering from IBS. In another study, nearly 35% of patients with IBS met diagnostic criteria for pelvic pain. This difference may be accounted for by difficulty in differentiating pelvic pain from abdominal pain. Patients with both IBS and pelvic pain were significantly more likely to have a history of childhood sexual abuse, hysterectomy, dysthymia, panic, and somatization disorders.

- **Premenstrual syndrome (PMS) and dysmenorrhea** are seen in approximately 10% of IBS patients. Other reports suggest rates as high as 50%. It appears that menstruation increases rectal sensitivity in IBS women compared to healthy volunteers (see Chapter 17). Fluctuations of prostaglandins or ovarian hormones may affect gut sensitivity and autonomic nervous system function. Other gynecologic pain syndromes that are associated less frequently with IBS include vaginitis (19%), amenorrhea (11%), and vulvodynia (9%).

- **Sexual function disturbances** range from 24% to 83% in a number of studies. More patients with IBS-C (49.4%) than patients with IBS-D (28%) report sexual dysfunction. Dyspareunia and abdominal pain during intercourse are the most common symptoms observed in female IBS patients. Decreased sexual drive was reported in 36.2% of men and 28.4% of women. These complaints appear to correlate with IBS symptom severity.

- **Urologic symptoms** such as frequency, urgency, and sensation of incomplete bladder evacuation are described in up to 50% of patients with IBS compared to healthy controls. In particular, interstitial cystitis, a syndrome characterized by bladder pain and increased urinary frequency, has been found in up to 30.2% of patients with IBS. There is no evidence for generalized smooth muscle disorder to explain the coexistence of these 2 disorders.

- **Miscellaneous** peripheral disorders reported to be associated with IBS include allergies (36%), chest pain (32%), dizziness/vertigo/syncope (22%), chronic cough (18%), asthma (13%), obesity (10%), and palpitations (5%).

Psychiatric Disorders[3-5]

Rates of depression and anxiety are higher in IBS patients, and these prevalence rates are intermediate between psychiatric populations and healthy controls. Psychological distress in IBS patients can usually be improved with appropriate treatment; however, patients who have personality disorders such as somatization or neuroticism are less responsive to treatment. Prospective studies have found that anxiety and depression are independent predictors of postinfectious IBS. Anxiety and depression also predict a poor outcome of IBS, including poor response to treatment. Overall, anywhere from 27% to 60% of patients with IBS are diagnosed with a psychiatric condition during their lifetime. The prevalence rates of psychiatric disorders vary depending upon the setting in which the IBS patient is seen; the rates are lower in the primary-care setting, approaching that of the general population, and are higher in the tertiary-care setting.

High frequency rates of sexual and physical abuse (30% to 56%) have been reported from many referral centers in the US and Europe in IBS patients compared with healthy controls. GI patients with abuse histories report greater psychological distress, more severe pain, greater impairment of functioning, and more healthcare seeking than GI patients without an abuse history.

- **Major depression** has been reported in up to 30.5% of IBS patients seen in an outpatient primary-care setting. Another smaller study found a 46% lifetime prevalence of major depression in 35 patients with IBS seen in a tertiary-care setting.

- **Generalized anxiety disorder** has been found in 26% to 34% of patients diagnosed with IBS and treated at a university-based medical center compared to 1% to 6% in healthy controls. Panic disorders are also highly correlated with IBS and have a lifetime prevalence of 26% to 31% as seen in a cohort of patients treated at a tertiary medical center.

- The prevalence of **post-traumaticstress disorder** (PTSD) is 34% in IBS patients seen at an urban academic medical center compared to 18% in non-IBS patients. Similar findings were seen in a study of IBS patients admitted to a clinical treatment center in whom 36% were diagnosed with PTSD.

- **Phobias** such as agoraphobia and social phobias have a reported lifetime prevalence of 20% and 34%, respectively, in IBS patients seen in a tertiary outpatient setting.

- **Substance abuse**, specifically alcohol abuse or dependence, has been described in up to 9% of IBS patients. One study of patients seeking outpatient treatment for alcohol abuse or dependence found a 42% prevalence of IBS.

- **Other psychological disorders** associated with IBS include somatization disorder (26%), hypochondriasis (9%), and obsessive-compulsive disorders (6% to 9%).

Summary

Nongastrointestinal disorders in IBS patients are common and pose additional hardship on their lives. In our practice, we take a careful history to identify these comorbid conditions. We try to educate our patients about how these disorders coexist and discuss the possible shared central processing of their symptoms originating from different parts of their bodies. We recognize that these patients may experience their symptoms more acutely, leading to a greater psychological distress. Therapeutically, we use a multidisciplinary approach to provide a clear, unified, and consistent treatment plan. For instance, a patient with IBS and fibromyalgia might be treated by a gastroenterologist, a rheumatologist, and a psychiatrist. Someone with IBS and pelvic pain may benefit from being seen by a gynecologist, a physical therapist specializing in pelvic floor disorders, a gastroenterologist, and a psychiatrist. We have found the greatest treatment success in patients who were motivated and involved in their care.

References

1. Ringel Y, Drossman DA, Whitehead WE, Naliboff BD, Mayer EA. Effect of abuse history on pain reports and brain responses to aversive visceral stimulation: An fMRI study. *Gastroenterology.* 2008;134:396-404.
2. Chang L. Brain responses to visceral and somatic stimuli in irritable bowel syndrome: a central nervous system disorder? *Gastroenterol Clin North Am.* 2005;34:271-279.
3. Whitehead WE, Palsson OS, Levy RR, et al. Comorbidity in irritable bowel syndrome. *Am J Gastroenterol.* 2007;102:2767-2776.
4. Whitehead WE, Palsson OS, Jones KR. Systematic review of the comorbidity of irritable bowel syndrome with other disorders: what are the causes and implications? *Gastroenterology.* 2002;122:1140-1156.
5. North CS, Hong BA, Alpers DH. Relationship of functional gastrointestinal disorders and psychiatric disorders: Implications for treatment. *World J Gastroenterol.* 2007;13(14):2020-2027.

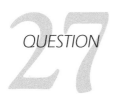

Is Fecal Incontinence More Common in Patients With IBS?

Kirsten T. Weiser, MD, MPH

Fecal incontinence (FI) is defined as the involuntary passage of fecal material or flatus after the successful completion of toilet training in early childhood. Fecal incontinence is often divided into major and minor subgroups, with minor incontinence described as the loss of flatus or a small amount of liquid stool, while major incontinence is defined as the loss of feces. Fecal incontinence is typically multifactorial, arising when propulsive forces of the stool overcome the resistive barriers of the anorectum. Stool consistency, bowel motility, rectal sensation, rectal compliance, completeness of evacuation, medications, and physical or cognitive abilities all may contribute to the development of fecal incontinence.

Not surprisingly, fecal incontinence is associated with a significant decrease in quality of life, decreased work productivity, depression, and social isolation. Fecal incontinence is one of the most common reasons for admission into nursing homes.

The prevalence of FI in the US population (age >50) is estimated to be 8.3% to 15.2%.[1] The prevalence is notably higher in certain populations, affecting up to 50% of the institutionalized elderly and up to 30% of women with urinary incontinence and pelvic organ prolapse. Historically, the male-to-female ratio for fecal incontinence was reported as 1:5. However, in recent population-based studies, men have a surprisingly high prevalence of FI (equal to that of women), suggesting that women are generally more likely to report fecal incontinence.[1] This also suggests that there is more to the development of fecal incontinence than obstetric injury alone. Common risk factors for the development of fecal incontinence, beyond obstetric injury, include postsurgical complications (eg, hemorrhoidectomy, lateral sphincterotomy), pelvic floor disorders, radiation injury, inflammatory bowel disease, spinal cord injury, cerebrovascular accident, and diabetes.[2]

Irritable bowel syndrome (IBS) has also been identified as an important risk factor for the development of fecal incontinence, particularly in IBS-diarrhea patients. In women over the age of 40 with IBS, the odds of having FI were 2.4 times that of healthy controls.[3] In part, this is due to the stool texture; loose stools and diarrhea have repeatedly been shown to increase the incidence of FI. In fact, for both men and women, having a loose or watery stool more frequently than 3 times per day was associated with a three- to fourfold increase in FI.[1] A recent study identified the development of fecal urgency as the main bowel-symptom predictor for new-onset FI.[4] Loose stools and stool frequency were also associated with FI but less so than the development of urgency.

Rectal hypersensitivity, common in IBS, has been associated with reduced rectal compliance and rectal hypercontractility.[4] Rectal hypersensitivity alone, however, has not clearly been shown to alter the number of incontinence events. This being said, rectal hypersensitivity has been shown to increase stool frequency (up to fourfold) and increase the degree of urgency leading to greater use of pads and restrictions on lifestyle. Furthermore, in a small study looking at patients with urgent fecal incontinence, nearly 100% of patients with FI had documented rectal hypersensitivity, when compared to controls. Additionally, these patients were also found to have increased colonic motility, in patterns similar to those seen in patients with IBS (unfortunately Rome III criteria were not applied to patients or controls).[5]

Treatment options for FI in patients with IBS are primarily designed to modify stool consistency and reduce colonic motility.[6] Dietary modifications such as altering fiber intake (usually a reduction in patients with loose stools) and removing excess caffeine or alcohol intake may improve stool form. Identification of missed lactose or fructose intolerance may further improve symptoms. The mainstay of medication therapy includes loperamide, a synthetic opioid that acts not only as an anti-diarrheal agent by decreasing colonic peristalsis but also by increasing sphincter tone and reducing urgency. Diphenoxylate, another opioid derivative, is another effective option but has two drawbacks when compared to loperamide: one, it crosses the blood-brain barrier and can thus cause mild euphoria; and two, it does not have the same effect on sphincter tone. Additional medication options include antispasmodics, which may reduce the gastrocolonic reflex and associated urgency to defecate. Low-dose tricyclic antidepressants may also reduce rectal hypersensitivity. Finally, biofeedback therapy is a well-described therapeutic intervention for fecal incontinence in general, though the specific utility in IBS patients with FI compared to other FI patients is not clear. While there is no single, standardized biofeedback program, generally, biofeedback training works to improve voluntary squeeze, modify anorectal sensation, and improve urge resistance training.

References

1. Whitehead WE, Borrud L, Goode PS, et al. Fecal incontinence in US adults: epidemiology and risk factors. *Gastroenterology.* 2009;137:512-517.
2. Varma G, Brown S, Creasman J, et al. Fecal incontinence in females older than aged 40 years: who is at risk? *Dis Colon Rectum.* 2006;49:841-851.
3. Chan CL, Scott M, Williams NS, Lunniss PJ. Rectal hypersensitivity worsens stool frequency, urgency, and lifestyle in patients with urge fecal incontinence. *Dis Colon Rectum.* 2005;48:134-140.
4. Rey E, Choung RS, Schleck CD, et al. Onset and risk factors for fecal incontinence in a US community. *Am J Gastroenterol.* 2010;105:412-419.
5. Roger CJ, Nicol L, Anderson JM, et al. Abnormal colonic motility: a possible association with urge fecal incontinence. *Dis Colon Rectum.* 2010;53:409-413.
6. Scarlett Y. Medical management of fecal incontinence. *Gastroenterology.* 2004;126(Suppl 1):S55-S63.

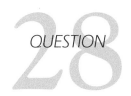

How Do I Evaluate and Treat Pelvic Floor Dysfunction in My Patients With IBS?

Adil E. Bharucha, MD, MBBS

In the context of functional bowel disorders, the term *pelvic floor dysfunction* encompasses disordered defecation, which can cause chronic constipation, and anal weakness, which can predispose to fecal incontinence in patients with diarrhea.[1-3] However, there is a wider spectrum of pelvic floor dysfunctions, characterized not only by anal but also rectal sensorimotor dysfunctions.[2] Moreover, while rectal evacuation disorders generally manifest as chronic constipation, they may also predispose to fecal incontinence. This chapter will focus on the assessment and management of defecatory disorders in patients with chronic constipation.

A comprehensive history of bowel habits, aided by pictorial stool form scales and if possible by bowel diaries, is essential because some symptoms (ie, anal digitation, sense of anal blockage during defecation, sense of incomplete evacuation after defecation) are more suggestive than others (eg, excessive straining, infrequent bowel habits, and hard stools) of disordered defecation.[4] In addition, while even healthy people may struggle to evacuate hard as opposed to soft stools, the inability to evacuate soft stools, and particularly liquid stools or enemas, strongly suggests disordered defecation. Not infrequently, irritable bowel syndrome (IBS) and pelvic floor dysfunction will coexist.[3]

A careful rectal examination is mandatory. Inspection may reveal anal fissures or large hemorrhoids in patients with pelvic floor dysfunction. Digital examination can assess anal pressure at rest, when patients contract or squeeze their anal sphincter and pelvic floor muscles, and during simulated evacuation. Normally, simulated evacuation is accompanied by relaxation of the anal sphincter and puborectalis muscle and perineal descent by 1 to 4 cm (Figure 28-1). Patients with defecatory disorders have one or more abnormal findings, including anismus (ie, high anal resting pressure), reduced or excessive perineal descent (ie, ballooning of the perineum), and/or rectal prolapse. The puborectalis may not relax normally, or paradoxically may contract, during simulated

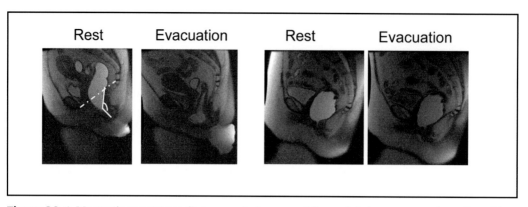

Figure 28-1. Magnetic resonance fluoroscopic images of the pelvis in an asymptomatic subject (left panel) and a patient with disordered defecation (right panel). The rectum was filled with ultrasound gel. In the asymptomatic subject, evacuation was accompanied by widening of the anorectal angle, indicated by an arc, and perineal descent by 4 cm relative to the pubococcygeal line, which is shown by a dotted line. In contrast, there was no perineal descent or change in the anorectal angle or rectal evacuation in the patient with disordered defecation (right panel).

evacuation. In my experience, relaxation of the puborectalis may not be perceptible even in patients with normal anorectal function. Therefore, except for patients who have paradoxical puborectalis contraction, abnormal perineal descent, particularly if markedly reduced or absent, is more useful than impaired puborectalis relaxation for identifying defecatory disorders.

While pelvic floor dysfunction can often be excluded or confirmed with reasonable confidence by a careful clinical assessment, anorectal testing is required because studies suggest that a clinical assessment alone does not suffice for identifying defecatory disorders.[5] Moreover, many patients are reassured by objective testing, and some insurance providers require an objective assessment before allowing the patient to proceed to pelvic floor retraining by biofeedback therapy. In most patients, anorectal manometry and a rectal balloon expulsion test suffice to confirm or exclude defecatory disorders. In selected circumstances (ie, when only one test is abnormal, when pelvic organ prolapse or a large rectocoele are suspected, or when there is a discrepancy between the clinical features and these anorectal tests), barium or magnetic resonance (MR) defecography is necessary to break the tie.[6]

The rectal balloon expulsion test is a very simple, sensitive, and specific test for diagnosing defecatory disorders. Patients are asked to expel a 4-cm rectal balloon filled with 50 mL of warm water while seated on a commode; normally, this requires less than 1 minute.[7] Alternatively, patients are asked to expel a rectal balloon, connected over a pulley to weights, in the left lateral decubitus position.[8] Depending on the technique, patients with pelvic floor dysfunction require more external traction or more time to expel the balloon. Perception of the desire to defecate is essential prior to normal defecation. Some patients with defecatory disorders have reduced rectal sensation.[9] While most laboratories inflate a rectal balloon by a standard volume, typically 50 mL, it has been suggested that when rectal sensation is reduced, patients may not perceive the desire to defecate at a volume of 50 mL, limiting their ability to evacuate the balloon even though rectal evacuation is preserved.[10] An alternative approach is to inflate the balloon by increasing volumes until patients experience the desire to defecate.[10] Further studies are necessary to compare these two techniques (ie, fixed versus variable balloon inflation) of assessing rectal evacuation.

Anal manometry may reveal a high anal resting pressure or anismus (ie, ≥90 mm Hg) in defecatory disorders.[6] A reduced recto-anal pressure gradient, expressed as the ratio or the difference between rectal and anal pressure, during simulated evacuation is also used to identify impaired rectal evacuation.[11] However, in our experience, this measure is not useful because many asymptomatic people also have an abnormal gradient during simulated evacuation.[12] Further studies to evaluate the utility of the recto-anal pressure gradient for identifying defecatory disorders are necessary. Except for Hirschsprung's disease, the recto-anal inhibitory reflex is preserved in chronic constipation.

Barium or MR defecography can identify structural abnormalities (eg, rectocele, enterocele, and rectal prolapse) and evaluate anorectal motion by measuring various parameters (ie, anorectal angle, perineal descent, anal diameter, puborectalis indentation, and rectal contents) at rest, during voluntary contraction, and during rectal evacuation.[13] Barium defecography should be performed with barium paste (eg, E-Z Paste, E-z-em Inc, Lake Success, NY) rather than liquid barium, and radiologists should be encouraged to measure anorectal parameters in addition to providing an overall impression. It can be challenging to measure these parameters because the bony landmarks necessary for making these measurements may not be clearly visible. MR defecography overcomes this limitation and, in contrast to barium defecography, does not entail radiation exposure and also visualizes bladder and urogenital prolapse. In a controlled study, MR defecography identified disturbances of evacuation and/or squeeze in 94% of patients with suspected defecation disorders.[8] In addition to examining the images, I also find it useful to review real-time images of the defecography.

While these anorectal tests are useful for identifying defecatory disorders, there are several caveats to interpreting test results. First, these tests may be abnormal even in asymptomatic people.[14,15] Second, the literature suggests that there is a relatively poor correlation among various tests (eg, anorectal manometry and defecography) in patients with defecatory disorders and that there is no true gold standard diagnostic test. Third, it is my perception that some patients with clinical features of pelvic floor dysfunction have seemingly normal rectal evacuation by testing, perhaps because they strain excessively to overcome increased pelvic floor resistance. Thus, an integrated assessment of clinical features and anorectal tests is necessary to confirm or exclude defecation disorders.

I manage defecatory disorders primarily by referring patients for pelvic floor retraining by biofeedback therapy, supplemented by laxatives and/or prokinetics as necessary to ensure stools are soft. Using electronically augmented feedback, patients are taught how to relax or contract muscles at appropriate times. Specifically, patients are educated about the normal physiology of defecation and errors in the manner they defecate. Then, they are taught how to strain appropriately (ie, increase intra-abdominal pressure) while ensuring that pelvic floor muscles, as evidenced by EMG activity or anal canal pressures, are relaxed. Subsequently, patients learn how to evacuate an air-filled balloon while the therapist assists by pulling on a catheter attached to the balloon. Some centers also include sensory training to teach the patient how to recognize weaker sensations of rectal filling. At Mayo Clinic, we provide two or three sessions daily over 2 weeks, primarily for patient convenience. Other centers provide 5 or 6 biweekly sessions lasting 30 to 60 minutes. Controlled studies show that pelvic floor retraining was superior to laxatives alone for improving symptoms and anorectal functions in defecatory disorders.[16,17] This improvement was sustained at 12 and 24 months. An abnormal rectal balloon expulsion test predicted the response to biofeedback therapy.[18]

There are several logistical challenges to providing biofeedback therapy for defecatory disorders. Many insurance programs do not cover pelvic floor retraining by biofeedback therapy for chronic constipation, but the situation is improving. While many therapists are familiar with Kegel exercises, biofeedback therapy for defecatory disorders is not widely available. Therapeutic options for patients who do not respond to biofeedback therapy are limited and unsatisfactory. While uncontrolled studies suggest that injection of botulinum toxin into the puborectalis muscle may be effective,[19] I have not found this useful in a small number of patients with defecatory disorders refractory to biofeedback therapy. An uncontrolled study suggests that sacral nerve stimulation may be effective. [20] Partial division of the puborectalis or anal sphincters can result in fecal incontinence and should not be considered for a functional disorder. After pelvic floor function improves, medically refractory constipation may be due to colonic motor dysfunction. In these patients, I assess colonic transit and, in selected cases, also colonic motor activity with a barostat-manometric assembly[21]; a subtotal colectomy may benefit patients who have colonic motor dysfunction but preserved pelvic floor function.

References

1. Bharucha AE. Pelvic floor: anatomy and function. *Neurogastroenterol Motil.* 2006;18(7):507-519.
2. Bharucha AE, Zinsmeister AR, Locke GR, et al. Risk factors for fecal incontinence: a population based study in women. *Am J Gastroenterol.* 2006;101:1305-1312.
3. Suttor VP, Prott GM, Hansen RD, Kellow JE, Malcolm A. Evidence for pelvic floor dyssynergia in patients with irritable bowel syndrome. *Dis Colon Rectum.* 2010;53(2):156-160.
4. Koch A, Voderholzer WA, Klauser AG, Muller-Lissner S. Symptoms in chronic constipation. *Dis Colon Rectum.* 1997;40(8):902-906.
5. Grotz RL, Pemberton JH, Talley NJ, Rath DM, Zinsmeister AR. Discriminant value of psychological distress, symptom profiles, and segmental colonic dysfunction in outpatients with severe idiopathic constipation. *Gut.* 1994;35(6):798-802.
6. Bharucha AE. Update of tests of colon and rectal structure and function. *J Clin Gastroenterol.* 2006;40(2): 96-103.
7. Rao SS, Hatfield R, Soffer E, Rao S, Beaty J, Conklin JL. Manometric tests of anorectal function in healthy adults. *Am J Gastroenterol.* 1999;94(3):773-783.
8. Bharucha AE, Fletcher JG, Seide B, Riederer SJ, Zinsmeister AR. Phenotypic variation in functional disorders of defecation. *Gastroenterology.* 2005;128:1199-1210.
9. Gladman MA, Lunniss PJ, Scott SM, Swash M. Rectal hyposensitivity. *Am J Gastroenterol.* 2006;101(5): 1140-1151.
10. Minguez M, Herreros B, Sanchiz V, et al. Predictive value of the balloon expulsion test for excluding the diagnosis of pelvic floor dyssynergia in constipation. *Gastroenterology.* 2004;126(1):57-62.
11. Bharucha AE, Wald A, Enck P, Rao S. Functional anorectal disorders. *Gastroenterology.* 2006;130(5): 1510-1518.
12. Ravi K, Zinsmeister AR, Bharucha AE. Do rectoanal pressures predict rectal balloon expulsion in chronic constipation? *Gastroenterology.* 2009;136(5):A101-102.
13. Bharucha AE. Update of tests of colon and rectal structure and function. *J Clin Gastroenterol.* 2006;40(2): 96-103.
14. Voderholzer WA, Neuhaus DA, Klauser AG, Tzavella K, Muller-Lissner SA, Schindlbeck NE. Paradoxical sphincter contraction is rarely indicative of anismus. *Gut.* 1997;41(2):258-262.
15. Freimanis MG, Wald A, Caruana B, Bauman DH. Evacuation proctography in normal volunteers. *Invest Radiol.* 1991;26(6):581-585.

16. Chiarioni G, Whitehead WE, Pezza V, Morelli A, Bassotti G. Biofeedback is superior to laxatives for normal transit constipation due to pelvic floor dyssynergia. *Gastroenterology.* 2006;130(3):657-664.

17. Rao SS, Seaton K, Miller M, et al. Randomized controlled trial of biofeedback, sham feedback, and standard therapy for dyssynergic defecation. *Clin Gastroenterol Hepatol.* 2007;5(3):331-338.

18. Chiarioni G, Salandini L, Whitehead WE. Biofeedback benefits only patients with outlet dysfunction, not patients with isolated slow transit constipation. *Gastroenterology.* 2005;129(1):86-97.

19. Maria G, Cadeddu F, Brandara F, Marniga G, Brisinda G. Experience with type A botulinum toxin for treatment of outlet-type constipation. *Am J Gastroenterol.* 2006;101(11):2570-2575.

20. Kamm MA, Dudding TC, Melenhorst J, et al. Sacral nerve stimulation for intractable constipation. *Gut.* 2010;59(3):333-340.

21. Ravi K, Bharucha AE, Camilleri M, Rhoten D, Bakken T, Zinsmeister AR. Phenotypic variation of colonic motor functions in chronic constipation. *Gastroenterology.* 2009;138(1):89-97.

SECTION V

TREATMENT FOR IBS

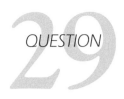

WHAT KEY EDUCATIONAL POINTS DO I NEED TO CONVEY TO MY PATIENTS WITH IBS?

Albena Halpert, MD

Patient education has been shown to decrease pain and anxiety, improve adherence to treatment, and enhance satisfaction with health care, thus reducing malpractice claims and health-care costs. Although the benefits of patient education are well recognized, many patients with irritable bowel syndrome (IBS) report that they are insufficiently informed about their condition and that physicians do not provide adequate education about their disorder.[1] The major barriers to effective IBS patient education include lack of time; poor or no reimbursement; the role of the biomedical model of illness, which emphasizes morphology and physiology and often overlooks the broader concept of illness experience; inadequate training of medical professionals in teaching skills; and lack of understanding or appreciation of the potential effectiveness of various educational approaches.

In the following section, I have highlighted key points related to the content and process of educating patients about IBS, and I have provided practical suggestions for their implementation in clinical practice.

The Process of Education Is as Important as the Factual Knowledge We Provide

Medical practice has traditionally adopted the pedagogical model of patient education, in which the physician, or "teacher," possesses medical skills and knowledge and is responsible for informing the patient about drug regimens, disease prognosis, or lifestyle modifications with patients contributing little other than a description of their illness. In many cases, patients may reject the information, overtly or covertly, due to personal concern, lack of understanding, or lack of agreement. In chronic disease, a partnership paradigm is emerging in which patients' expertise is similar in importance to the expertise of professionals. This paradigm implies that, while professionals are experts about diseases, patients are experts about their own lives. Whereas traditional patient education offers information and technical skills, self-management education teaches problem-solving skills. Sometimes called "patient empowerment," this concept holds that patients accept responsibility for managing their own conditions and are encouraged to solve their own problems with information.[1]

CLINICAL IMPLICATIONS

- Accept and respect each patient as a person—be trusting, understanding, respectful, and nonjudgmental.
- The patient can only learn to the extent that he or she is ready to learn.
- Use patients' prior experience as an opportunity to teach. *"What has worked for you before?"*
- Concentrate on daily life disease problem-solving rather than talking in general terms; consider the use of action plans. *"What can you do if you are at work and your stomach starts to hurt?"*
- Help the patient develop criteria and methods for measuring progress. *"What will be the best way for you to keep track of how you are doing?"*

Eliciting Patients' Prior Knowledge about IBS/ Conceptions and Misconceptions Is Critical to Effective Education

Knowledge is thought to be stored in the form of "conceptions" that are coherent identifiable ideas incorporating information, values, and beliefs. Learning occurs when existing conceptions change through the addition of new ideas and/or clarification of old ones and/or exchange of misconceptions for better ones. If a person does not find a new idea compelling, he or she rejects it, and no learning takes place. Unless preconceptions are identified, learning may be blocked, because existing conceptions affect what, and how, people learn.

CLINICAL IMPLICATIONS

- Start with finding out patients' educational needs: *What do you know about IBS? What would you like to know about IBS the most?*
- To introduce and successfully negotiate new ideas, first identify the gaps, confusion, and errors in patients' conceptions. For example, when introducing the idea of using antidepressants for the treatment of IBS, the clinician may ask, *"What do you think about this?"* This approach allows for the identification of any barriers to taking centrally acting agents, for example, the patient's concern of, *"Am I going to be addicted to them?"*
- If a specific concern such as this one is not addressed, it is unlikely the patient will take the medication.

Many Patients Hold Misconceptions Regarding IBS Mortality and Morbidity, Which May Contribute to Unnecessary Worrying

Research findings indicate that many IBS patients mistakenly believe that IBS can lead to cancer, colitis, or malnutrition; shorten their life; or require surgery.[2] Correcting these misconceptions reduces disease-related anxiety and improves patients' satisfaction with their visit and may possibly reduce future health-care utilization.

CLINICAL IMPLICATIONS

- Inquire about specific IBS-related concerns and worries, and then address them.
- Patients may not volunteer this information unless asked directly.
- Examples:
  - *"What about your condition concerns you or worries you?"*
  - *"Many patients worry that IBS may become cancer, cause colitis, shorten one's life, or require surgery. We know that IBS is not associated with any of these conditions."*

Address Patients' Specific Questions/Educational Needs Regarding IBS Rather Than Provide General Information About the Condition

If there are several questions, prioritize (with the patient) those you plan to address during the visit. The most common topics patients are interested in learning about, in order of ranked importance based on a national survey on patient educational needs,[3] are outlined in Table 29-1. Suggested sample explanations are also included.

Take into Consideration Patients' Health Literacy Level and Motivation to Learn and Adjust Your Teaching Style

Health literacy is defined as a patient's ability to obtain, process, and understand basic health information and services needed to make appropriate health decisions. Health literacy is a better predictor of one's health status than age, income, employment, ethnicity, or education level. It is important to realize that nearly one-half (47%) of adults in the United States read below an 8th grade level. Many health-care providers are unaware of the large number of patients in their practices who have limited health literacy. In addition, most patients forget up to 80% of what their doctor tells them as soon as they leave the office, and nearly 50% of what they do remember is recalled incorrectly. By using clear health communication techniques, you can help your patients better understand and manage their condition.

Table 29-1

Topics That Most Interest IBS Patients[3]

Topics	Suggested Explanations & Notes for the Clinician
What foods should I avoid?	*"There is no specific IBS diet. Often eating rather than specific food can trigger an attack. Eating small, frequent meals vs few large meals may be helpful. Keeping a 2- to 3-week food diary may show potential triggers for a specific patient (e.g., fatty meals, milk products, nuts)."*
	Note Discourage overly restrictive diets. Lactose intolerance is common in patients with IBS. Consider dairy-free diet for 2 weeks to determine if there is lactose intolerance or perform hydrogen breath test to evaluate for lactose intolerance. Consider fructose intolerance and celiac sprue. Refer to a dietitian when appropriate/available.
What causes IBS?	*"IBS is the most common GI disorder. In IBS, the bowel looks normal but its function is altered in several ways: 1) Increased gut sensitivity (lower threshold for pain). 2) Altered brain-gut regulation (abnormal brain-gut "wiring") and 3) Abnormal motility (the ability of the gut to squeezes and relax). Stress can make IBS worse but does not cause it. IBS is a real GI condition and it is "not in your head." There is no specific test to confirm the condition and, thus, a "negative test" does not mean there is no real disease."*
Coping strategies to reduce symptoms	*"It is important to realize that IBS symptoms can cause stress, but similarly, the way you respond to the symptoms (deal with the illness) can make symptoms better or worse. Therefore, it is very important not only to treat the specific symptoms (eg, pain, bloating, and diarrhea) but also to be aware of your own response to having symptoms. Specific strategies to improve coping may be helpful, such as relaxation techniques, at the onset of symptoms, expressive writing (e.g., keeping a diary), using your social support, or getting professional help. For example, a psychologist may be able to help you work on specific coping strategies. Treatment of anxiety or depression, if present, can result in significant improvement in IBS symptoms, because of the close connection between the brain and the gut."*
Medication to prevent attack	Note The responses to medications differ between specific clinical presentations and among people. Consider: a) frequency and severity of attacks; b) IBS-related quality of life; and c) presence of psychiatric co-morbidity when choosing a pharmacological agent (eg, antispasmodics given as needed vs daily antidepressant). Also consider alternative medicines or nonpharmacological approaches (eg, relaxation techniques) alone or in combination with medications.

continued

<u>Table 29-1 Continued</u>

Topics That Most Interest IBS Patients[3]

Topics	Suggested Explanations & Notes for the Clinician
Will my IBS ever go away/get better?	*"IBS symptoms are usually chronic (come and go) and may improve with age, particularly in women."*
Psychological factors in IBS	*"Are there any other factors that can worsen your symptoms, like diet, physical activity, or stress?"*
	Note In addition to obtaining potentially meaningful clinical information, asking patients a question like this conveys a high level of acceptance of stress being one of many factors that may trigger IBS rather than IBS being a "psychiatric" problem.
Research Studies Available	Potential sources of information on ongoing clinical studies include: local universities and web sites (www.iffgd.org, www.clinicaltrials.gov).
What are normal/ abnormal bowel habits?	*"Having between three bowel movements a day to three a week is considered normal. It is OK not to have a bowel movement every day or have several bowel movements a day. Change from what is normal for you is more important than the actual number of bowel movements."*
What causes bloating?	*"Several factors may contribute to bloating in patients with IBS, such as decreased rate of passing gas or swallowing too much air. Sometimes there are too many bacteria in the small bowel producing gas."*
Is IBS going to shorten my life?	*"IBS will not shorten your life."*

CLINICAL IMPLICATIONS

Consider using the following 4 simple techniques:

1. Check for comprehension with the "Teach Back" method: *"I want to be sure that I did a good job explaining how to take your medications, because this can be confusing. Can you tell me how will you take the medication?"* or *"Just to be sure we are on the same page, why don't you tell me what you would do when …"*

If your patient is not able to repeat the information accurately, try to re-phrase rather than just repeat the information and check for understanding again.

2. Use visual aids and illustrations. Many people remember information better when it is presented to them visually. You can draw simple pictures or diagrams to help explain your instructions. An excellent source of patient information is the International Foundation for Functional Gastrointestinal Disorders web site (www. iffgd.org). Other sources are listed in the reference section.

3. Avoid using words with multiple meanings; avoid using idioms (eg, "feeling blue") and acronyms (eg, CAT scan)

4. Consider giving each patient a checklist or "action plan" outlining a mutual treatment plan.

What Every Patient With IBS Needs to Know

Patient education is most effective when it is individualized to a patient's specific needs. Therefore, it is not possible to design a script that will be helpful for all IBS patients. Below are the key educational points that will benefit most patients with IBS:

- IBS is a real gastrointestinal condition (not "in your head") that can significantly affect one's life. (This provides validation and demonstrates empathy.)

- IBS is a chronic medical condition, though the symptoms can come and go. There is no magic pill for IBS. (This helps patients set realistic expectations.)

- There are many things we can do to make it better and help you manage it. You may have long periods of time (years for some patients) without experiencing any symptoms. (This provides hope to the patient, which is essential.)

- IBS does not cause cancer, colitis, or any other problems. It does not shorten your life. (This helps to clarify potential misconceptions.)

- For some people with IBS, stress can trigger their symptoms or make them worse. (This can be used to explore the role of psychological factors in IBS.)

- We need to work in partnership/together to help you manage your IBS. (This emphasizes the need for a collaborative approach.)

References

1. Lorig K. *Patient Education: A Practical Approach*. Thousand Oaks, CA: Sage Publications, Inc; 2001.
2. Lacy BE, Weiser K, Noddin L, et al. Irritable bowel syndrome: patients' attitudes, concerns and level of knowledge. *Aliment Pharmacol Ther*. 2007;25:1329-1341.
3. Halpert A, Dalton C, Palsson O, et al. What patients know about irritable bowel syndrome (IBS) and what they would like to know? National survey on patient educational needs in IBS and development and validation of the patient educational needs questionnaire (PEQ). *Am J Gastroenterol*. 2007;102:1972-1982.

Sources of Additional Patient Information on IBS

International Foundation for Functional Gastrointestinal Disorders (IFFGD)—www.iffgd.org
National Library of Medicine—www.nlm.nih.gov/medlineplus/healthtopics.html
National Institute of Diabetes and Digestive and Kidney Diseases—www.niddk.nih.gov
The American Gastroenterological Association—www.gastro.org
The American College of Gastroenterology—www.acg.gi.org

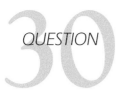
WHAT DIETARY RECOMMENDATIONS SHOULD I MAKE TO MY PATIENTS WITH IBS?

Christine L. Frissora, MD, FACG, FACP

Irritable bowel syndrome (IBS) is like ice cream. It comes in a wide spectrum of colors and flavors. In my practice, which focuses on patients with functional gastrointestinal disorders, I tell my patients that although many IBS patients have similar symptoms, all patients are unique in why their symptoms developed and how their symptoms are expressed. Although we now have a much better explanation for why IBS develops in some patients (see Chapters 13 and 14), the truth is that we clearly do not understand all of the etiologic factors that lead to the development of IBS. In addition, we are now aware of a number of different disorders that have symptoms that are quite similar to those expressed by those patients who clearly have IBS. Stated another way, a number of medical conditions tend to masquerade as IBS. Thus, some patients have been mistakenly diagnosed with IBS when in fact their symptoms actually represent celiac disease, a food intolerance, a food sensitivity, a gastrointestinal parasite, pelvic floor dysfunction, or a preservative sensitivity.

One inherent problem with IBS is that symptoms of IBS are nonspecific. Thus, symptoms of lower abdominal discomfort with loose stools may represent a true and accurate diagnosis of IBS. However, these same symptoms could also represent lactose intolerance, fructose intolerance, celiac disease, or a reaction to a medication. In my practice, I spend a large amount of time during the initial interview taking a careful dietary history to help identify those disorders that may mimic IBS, because the treatment will obviously be completely different. A thorough medical history, including prior abdominal surgeries (especially prior cholecystectomy or surgery to the colon and small intestine), diet, travel, medication use (including birth control pills), the use of dietary supplements and alternative medications, and the use of probiotics is essential in order to make the correct diagnosis and initiate the proper treatment. Some of the questions I like to ask my patients include the following:

- What medications do you take?
- What supplements do you take?
- What vitamins do you take?
- What probiotics do you take?
- What herbal remedies do you take?
- What health foods do you eat?

You will be amazed at the plethora of "healthy, all-natural" substances patients take that, unknowingly, can cause significant problems. I also ask patients specifically about "sugar-free" candy or "dietetic" breath mints, chewing gum, and breath fresheners. The diabetic patient with "autonomic dysfunction," the ballerina, or the bride-to-be trying to lose weight may be overdosing on Stevia or other artificial sweeteners. Ask patients to bring in everything and look at the labels together. You may be shocked at what is contained in a supposedly healthy food or supplement. Sometimes, a step as simple as changing from a name brand to a generic birth control pill could be enough to trigger bloating, nausea, or discomfort.

In essence, a lot of what we eat makes us sick. I like to think of food as medicine. Remind your patients that you are what you eat, and remind them to read food and medication labels carefully. I strongly believe that most Americans eat too much junk food and too much processed food. The American diet is high in omega-6 fats, which can clog arteries, alter brain function, and do unknown things to the intestinal tract. As an example of how diet can cause symptoms in the GI tract, during the past few decades, the incidence of celiac disease has been on the rise, possibly due in part to the processed and hydrolyzed gluten we consume. I firmly believe that we all need to detoxify ourselves from toxic foods and chemicals, whether this is specifically to improve IBS symptoms or to improve our general physical and mental health. For my patients, I emphasize the following: focus on fresh fruits and vegetables; avoid overeating; realize that water stored in plastic bottles is potentially loaded with toxins and possibly even carcinogens; avoid processed foods, canned foods, and preservatives; and use organic foods when available. In addition, for my patients who do not know how to cook, I ask them to learn. Not only will they save money, but they will also lose inches around the waistline and reduce hours spent with symptoms of lower abdominal gas and bloating. I tell patients to focus on cooked vegetables with soluble fiber (acorn squash, butternut squash, yams, carrots, root vegetables), fruits (avocado, peaches, berries), certain whole grains (organic oats), and certain dairy products (organic milk).

During our office visit, I also ask my IBS patients to try to avoid animal products. Overconsumption of animal proteins and animal fats may cause cancer, arteriosclerosis, osteoporosis, obesity, high cholesterol, diabetes, and high blood pressure. Overconsumption of meat has been associated with a variety of problems, including liver, lung, kidney, nervous system, and reproductive disorders, birth defects, and miscarriages. Additionally, the animals that we eat are often fed antibiotics, steroids, and growth hormones, and they are often sprayed directly with chemical fertilizers, pesticides, insecticides, and herbicides. This cannot be safe for your patients in the long run. Meat, seafood, and dairy may also contain BHC, DDT, chlordane, linden, dioxin, dieldrin, and heptachlor. Some fish contain high levels of contaminants, pesticide residues, pollutants, and additional toxins, such as mercury and PCBs. High levels of mercury cause disrupted immune function, blindness, paralysis, high blood pressure, reduction in fertility and virility, and increased risk for cardiac mortality. These toxins and carcinogens disrupt all of our bodily functions, including our bowel system and metabolism.

Last, do not forget that there are hidden preservatives in the diet that can trigger IBS symptoms. Some are obvious—aspartame may cause dyspeptic symptoms, and sorbitol may cause cramping and diarrhea. However, there are hidden preservatives that can irritate the GI tract, too. For example, consider monosodium glutamate (MSG). MSG is commonly added to many prepared foods during the manufacturing process. MSG can react with other foods, and the ensuing reaction creates free glutamic acid, which can cause GI distress. Remind your patients to read food labels carefully, as MSG may not specifically be mentioned. In addition, note that the following substances may contain MSG-like substances: autolyzed yeast, caseinate, carageenan, gelatin, glutamic acid (glutamate), maltodextrin, monopotassium glutamate, pectin, protease, protein fortified ingredients, soy protein, textured vegetable protein, whey protein. The FDA considers labels such as "no MSG" or "no added MSG" to be misleading if the food contains ingredients that are sources of free glutamate, such as hydrolyzed protein.

What specific recommendations do I give my patients? Over the years, I have assembled a list of suggestions, which are summarized in Figure 30-1.

Vitamins

Please consult with your physician before beginning any supplement or vitamin.

- Vitamin C loosens the stool; if you are constipated, 500 to 1000 mg of vitamin C with dinner may help. Remember that vitamin C can cause reflux and esophagitis so it should not be taken late at night just before going to bed.
- Bring the exact bottle or label with you to the doctor so he or she can see exactly what is in the product you are taking.
- Beware of "natural remedies." Some of the advertising is false, and some products are contaminated with substances that can cause pancreatitis or kidney or liver disease.
- Just because something is "natural" does not mean it is safe or effective.
- Beware of "colon cleansers." They contain medications like "natural" sienna, and your colon can become tolerant to these medications and require ever-increasing doses.
- Do not take vitamins first thing in the morning. Take all *medically necessary* vitamins later in the day. Many patients note significant GI distress after consuming a cup of coffee, orange juice, and a large multivitamin first thing in the morning.
- Olive oil and mineral oil both loosen the stool. Olive oil is fattening, and mineral oil is not. Olive oil tastes good, while mineral oil does not. Use mineral oil if you are heavy and trying to lose weight, and use olive oil if you are thin. You can put either oil in your salad dressing (remember to shake it well). If you have symptoms of IBS with constipation, 1 to 4 tablespoons with dinner, on salad or cooked vegetables like acorn squash or chopped spinach, will lead to a softer bowel movement the following morning. Caution: remind your patients not to swallow mineral oil by itself, especially in the evening, as people can aspirate it.

DR. FRISSORA'S DIET FOR THE SENSITIVE STOMACH

"What Can I Eat, Doctor?"
This is meant to be a general guideline and will vary with each patient.
If you have CELIAC DISEASE or SPRUE, avoid wheat, barley, rye, and their derivatives.

Usually Tolerated
(in moderation)

Soluble fiber
oatmeal, berries, beets, cooked lentils, legumes, split pea soup, chickpeas, peas, carrots, yams, peaches, blueberries, strawberries, grits, Cream of Wheat, papaya, mango, kiwi

Organic yogurt [Greek: Total, Stonyfield]

Fish, shrimp

Rice, pasta, couscous, noodles, pastina

Egg whites

Lentil soup

Homemade chicken soup, dumplings

Banana, plantain, polenta

Cornflakes, Rice Krispies, Special K

Chamomile & herbal teas

Nectarines, apricots

Watermelon, honeydew, cantaloupe

Avocado, olive oil

Udon noodle soup, tender, cooked baby spinach

Graham crackers

Broccoli and cauliflower (tolerated best in a puree soup)

Cooked mashed rutabaga, turnip, parsnip

Homemade vegetable soup

Waffles, pancakes, mashed potatoes

Crackers
Low-salt Wheat Thins, rice crackers, unsalted Saltines

Baby leaf/red leaf lettuce in small amounts

Stewed, tender meat, Beef Bourguignonne

Small pieces of cooked carrots, celery, zucchini with rice, pasta and couscous

Use Caution

Citrus & tomato

"Diet" sugar-free products

Alcohol

Grapes

Chocolate (constipating)

Raw broccoli

Raw cauliflower

Cabbage

Cole slaw

Cold cuts

Iceberg lettuce

Popcorn

Dairy

Caffeine

Cheese (bloat)

Lactose

Avoid

Crude fiber (residue):
Eggplant skin, bell peppers, cucumber skin

MSG (pain & diarrhea)

Large seeds, husks

Nuts

Potato skins

Spicy food, curry

Fried foods, fats

Carbonated beverages

High-fructose corn syrup

Snapple, Gatorade

Garlic, onions

All artificial sweeteners:
Splenda, Equal,
Sweet'N Low

Diet soda

Sugar-free gum & candy

Zone bars, Power bars

Green tea

Hints:
• **Chew well**
• **Eat 6 small meals a day**
• **Use chewable vitamins**
• **Drink liquids between meals**
• **Eat slowly**

Figure 30-1. Dr. Frissora's Diet for the Sensitive Stomach.

Prenatal Vitamins and Iron

If you are a healthy man or postmenopausal woman, you probably do not need iron, but if you do, this is my advice:

• I recommend prenatal multivitamins for patients who need iron (menstruating or pregnant women) because they are rich in other nutrients like B vitamins (for stress!) and other things that help the hair, skin and nails.

    a. Duet DHA (which contains ferrazone as the iron, a vegetarian omega-3 source, and a low dose of docusate) helps constipation. One after dinner or before bed should loosen stool the following morning.

    b. Prenate elite is the most constipating prenatal vitamin. One after dinner will make the stool more formed.

- Slow Fe is generally a well-tolerated iron supplement.
- Chewable Flintstones vitamins with iron are also well tolerated after dinner but contain an artificial sweetener that can have a laxative-type effect.

Calcium Supplements

- Calcium may be important in regulating body fat and possibly to prevent colon cancer, but if you have kidney stones or parathyroid disease, calcium can be dangerous. Always ask your doctor before taking calcium or any other supplement.
- Calcium can cause bloating. The chewable form is usually better than tablets.
- Calcium supplements that contain magnesium or zinc can cause loose stools. This would be good for someone who is constipated but is not good for someone who has diarrhea.
- If you are constipated and need calcium, use CaMgZn by CVS natural or Posture D.
- If you have diarrhea and need calcium, use Oscal
- If you have reflux and need calcium, suck on three or four Tums each day.
- It appears that calcium and vitamin D best serve the bones when they are taken together. The stomach will handle this best about an hour after lunch or dinner.
- The importance of exercise, building core body strength, and weight lifting in moderation cannot be underestimated.

Artificial Sweeteners

- I believe that artificial sweeteners of all kinds should be avoided.
- The alternative sweeteners often used in "sugar-free chocolate," like sorbitol and mannitol, cause diarrhea and bloating.
- If you take liquid medications, they may contain artificial sweeteners as well. For example, NutraSweet, Splenda, and Equal can all cause nausea and dyspepsia (upper abdominal discomfort).
- High fructose corn syrup, a sweetener added to many foods and beverages in the United States, can cause bloating and diarrhea.
- Check all labels, especially "light" yogurt. They commonly have artificial sweeteners in them.

Probiotics

- Probiotics are not well understood yet.
- Some probiotics can cause bloating or nausea. When you swallow a billion bacteria,

you can expect gas and bloating. The two I have found most useful for the treatment of IBS are:

+ *Saccharomyces boulardii* (Florastor)—250 mg twice a day for diarrhea (taken 30 minutes before a meal). In addition, this may be helpful to treat or prevent antibiotic-associated diarrhea and "*C difficile* colitis."

+ Align (*Bifidobacterium*) can help gas, bloating, and urgency.

• Try not to spend a fortune on "natural" remedies. A lot of them do not have any safety or efficacy data to support their use.

+ Probiotics cannot be given to immunocompromised people. If you have cancer, AIDS, or are taking prednisone or 6-MP, you should not take probiotics.

+ Yogurts like Activia (with added probiotics) can actually be too strong for some patients, while it can help others with IBS.

Miscellaneous

• Antihistamine medications, including Benadryl, may be constipating.

• If you are suffering from chronic constipation, consider whether your antihistamine medications might be contributing to it.

Foods That Improve Diarrhea

• Bananas, white rice, rice crackers, rice milk, white meat chicken

• Pedialyte for rehydration (not Gatorade—it is too high in fructose)

• Isomil DF (a binding infant formula with calories)

• *Saccharomyces boulardii* (Florastor), an effective "probiotic" for diarrhea. Take one a day before lunch.

Foods That Improve Constipation

• Five servings a day of foods such as berries, pears, peaches, plums, papaya, mango, kiwi, raisins, prunes, prune juice (if not too gassy), chick peas, carrots, celery, snap peas, snow peas (eat the pod), green beans, yellow wax beans, acorn squash/butternut squash with olive oil.

• Five glasses of water or herbal decaffeinated tea; more if you can.

• Avoid foods and supplements that improve diarrhea (see above).

Things That Cause Bloat or GI Distress

• Many probiotics cause bloating (*Saccharomyces boulardii* does not)

• Cheese

• All carbonated beverages: beer, soda, and seltzer included

• All artificial sweeteners (Splenda, Equal, aspartame, sorbitol, etc)

- Zone bars, Power bars
- Green tea can cause nausea in some patients
- High fructose corn syrup (Activia yogurt, Snapple, Gatorade, and many prepared foods)
- Onions, garlic
- MSG and similar agents (carneengan, monoammonium glutamate, gelatin, caseinate, hydrolyzed protein)

Foods in General

- Cooked foods always go down easier, so if you want to eat a lot of vegetables, home-made soup is best; chew all food as well as you can. If you don't have a Crock pot, get one, because stewed vegetables and meats go down easier than barbeque, broiled, or fried.
- Homemade foods are easier to control than restaurant food.
- Watch out for sodium and MSG derivatives present in soups and even "natural" chicken broth.
- Animal products in general are contaminated with bacteria and hormones. Avoid them if you can.

References

1. Shepherd SJ, Parker FC, Muir JG, Gibson PR. Dietary triggers of abdominal symptoms in patients with irritable bowel syndrome: randomized, placebo-controlled evidence. *Clin Gastroenterol Hepatol.* 2008;6:765-771.
2. Choi YK, Kraft N, Zimmerman B, et al. Fructose intolerance in IBS and utility of fructose-restricted diet. *J Clin Gastroenterol.* 2008;42:233-238.
3. Skoog SM, Bharucha AE, Zinsmeister AR. Comparison of breath testing with fructose and high fructose corn syrups in health and IBS. *Neurogastroenterol Motil.* 2008;20:505-511.
4. Goldstein R, Braverman D, Stankiewicz H. Carbohydrate malabsorption and the effect of dietary restriction on symptoms of irritable bowel syndrome and functional bowel complaints. *Isr Med Assoc J.* 2000;2:583-587.
5. Evans PR, Piesse C, Bak YT, Kellow JE. Fructose-sorbitol malabsorption and symptom provocation in irritable bowel syndrome: relationship to enteric hypersensitivity and dysmotility. *Scand J Gastroenterol.* 1998;33:1158-1163.

Acknowledgment: I would like to thank Sarah T. Rodeo for content, fact checking, and editorial assistance.

WHAT IS THE RELATIONSHIP BETWEEN FRUCTOSE INTOLERANCE AND IBS?

Fernando Fernández-Bañares, MD, PhD

Malabsorption of sugars (lactose, fructose, and/or sorbitol) from a normal diet may induce chronic abdominal discomfort in sensitive individuals, including abdominal distension, flatulence, cramps, and diarrhea. There may be an intrasubject and intersubject variability in the threshold leading to gastrointestinal distress after ingestion of incompletely absorbed carbohydrates.[1] Whether sugar malabsorption will cause symptoms depends on several factors besides the absorptive capacity, such as the quantity and quality of the ingested carbohydrate load, the time spent to consume, and the nature of concomitant meals. Other factors additionally implicated include the rate of gastric emptying, the response of the small intestine to an osmotic load, small intestinal and colonic motility, the metabolic capacity of the colonic bacterial microflora, and the compensatory capacity of the colon to reabsorb water and short-chain fatty acids.[2]

Dietary sugars can be naturally present in foods (such as fructose in fruit or lactose in milk) or added to the food. In the past few decades, there has been an increased intake of simple sugars in processed foods and soft drinks.[3] The consumption of fructose has increased greatly in the United States as a result of increased use of high fructose corn syrups (HFCS) in soft drinks and confectionery. According to recent estimates in the US population, the mean consumption of fructose is 54.7 g/day, being higher in adolescents (73 g/day).[4] This translates into 43 to 60 pounds of high fructose corn syrup per person each year, an increase of almost 50% in the past 2 decades.[5] On the other hand, sorbitol is the most consumed sugar alcohol. Small amounts of sorbitol are present in some fruits of the *Rosaceae* family (apples, pears, cherries, apricots, and plums), but its content in certain sugar-free sweet foods may be considerable.[6] Sorbitol is also used as an additive for purposes other than sweetening in foods and medicine (many liquid medications), as a consequence of its unique combination of functional properties as a humectant, bulking agent, stabilizer, softener, emulsifier, and its surface-active properties.

The presence of fructose malabsorption, even in a patient with an organic abdominal disease, cannot be considered pathologic per se. In fact, the prevalence of fructose *plus* sorbitol malabsorption is similar in both healthy populations and IBS patients.[7-9] So, fructose-sorbitol malabsorption would be regarded as a "physiologic" event, with a role in promoting the growth of colonic microflora, as do other fermentable, poorly absorbed carbohydrates. However, as will be argued in this chapter, restricting fructose-sorbitol intake may improve intestinal symptoms in a subset of IBS patients.

Diagnosis of Fructose Malabsorption

There are some unresolved questions regarding the diagnosis of fructose malabsorption using breath hydrogen testing.[10] The most important issue is that it is unclear what the optimal dosage of fructose is to detect clinically meaningful malabsorption. Incomplete absorption after a 50-g fructose load was observed in 37.5% (10% solution) and 71% (20% solution) of healthy people.[11] It has been suggested that a dose of 25 g (10% solution) more closely approaches daily intake, and in pediatrics a dose of 1 g/kg has been recommended.[10] However, it is of great importance to recognize that simultaneous ingestion of glucose *increases* fructose absorption,[1] and the majority of dietary sources of fructose also contain glucose.[1,6] On the other hand, simultaneous ingestion of sorbitol interferes with the absorption of fructose, and coingestion of fructose and sorbitol is likely to be frequent.[12] Therefore, breath testing of fructose alone probably does not reflect fructose absorption in everyday life, making interpretation of the test extremely unreliable from a clinical point of view.[13] In this situation, the coadministration of fructose *plus* sorbitol may be a more consistent approach to the problem.[12] The prevalence of fructose *plus* sorbitol malabsorption in IBS is similar to that in healthy controls; however, IBS patients experienced significantly more symptoms than healthy subjects after fructose *plus* sorbitol malabsorption,[7-9] whereas there were no differences when fructose or sorbitol was administered alone.[8] Thus, some authors prefer to assess malabsorption of a fructose *plus* sorbitol mixture instead of malabsorption of fructose alone. For that, a mixture of fructose (20 g) and sorbitol (3.5 g) has been proposed.[12]

Fructose-Sorbitol Malabsorption and IBS

As mentioned, sugar malabsorption induced significantly more symptoms in patients with IBS than in healthy subjects.[7-9,14] In the only controlled study published to date, more severe symptoms were observed after intake of a fructose-sorbitol mixture than after the intake of sucrose (as a control well-absorbed solution), in patients with diarrhea-predominant IBS. In addition, lactulose administration, a nonabsorbable carbohydrate, induced more symptoms in IBS patients than in healthy controls.[8]

In unblinded, uncontrolled observational studies, 40% to 75% of IBS patients reported substantial improvement in symptoms after restriction of malabsorbed sugar(s) (ie, lactose, fructose, and/or sorbitol).[6,9,15-19] Whether this therapeutic effect represents a specific result of the sugar restricted diet or whether improvements seen represent no more than a placebo effect needs to be further assessed in controlled studies. A fructose restricted diet has been shown to improve mood and depressive symptoms in fructose malabsorbers[20]; because depressive symptoms are frequent in IBS patients, this mechanism may explain sustained improvement of both gastrointestinal and mood symptoms in some patients.

Table 31-1

Natural Foods With Moderate to High Fructose Content Expressed as Total Fructose, Total Glucose, and as Fructose in Excess of Glucose

Food	Average Serving	Glucose (g)	Fructose (g)	Excess Fructose (g)
Watermelon	1 slice, 100 g	0.99	1.32	0.33
Pineapple	1 slice, 85 g	1.25	1.7	0.45
Orange	1 slice, 140 g	2.08	2.33	0.25
Cantaloupe	1 slice, 100 g	1.44	2.1	0.66
Custard apple	1 piece, 170 g	12.4	13.5	1.1
Honey	1 tablespoon	6.8	8.2	1.4
Mandarin	1 serving, 170 g	2.59	3.4	1.8
Peach	1 piece, 140 g	1.16	2.76	1.9
Carambola	1 piece, 85 g	0.86	2.76	1.9
Pear	1 piece, 100 g	3.77	6.31	2.54
Mango	1 piece, 200 g	1.85	5.95	4.1
Apple	1 piece, 150 g	3.78	9.17	5.9

Modified from Fernández-Bañares F, Rosinach M, Esteve M, et al. Sugar malabsorption in functional abdominal bloating: A pilot study on the long-term effect of dietary treatment. *Clin Nutr.* 2006;25:824-831 and Barret JS, Gibson PR. Clinical ramifications of malabsorption of fructose and other short-chain carbohydrates. *Practical Gastroenterology.* 2007;31:51-65.

Recently, the effects on gastrointestinal symptoms of a carbohydrate-restricted diet were evaluated in a randomized, double-blind, quadruple-arm, crossover, placebo-controlled, rechallenge trial in patients with IBS and fructose malabsorption who had previously improved with a diet low in poorly absorbed short-chain carbohydrates and sugar alcohols (Fermentable Oligosaccharides, Disaccharides, Monosaccharides, and Polyols: the FODMAP diet).[21] Frequency and severity of overall and individually evaluated symptoms were significantly and markedly higher for free fructose, fructans, or the mixture than for control glucose. Symptoms were induced in a dose-dependent manner and mimicked previous IBS symptoms. Results of this study provide evidence that fructose and fructans are dietary triggers for symptoms suggestive of IBS when fructose malabsorption is present and suggest that the efficacy is due to restriction of poorly absorbed short-chain carbohydrates, in general, and not to a placebo effect.

Fructose- and Sorbitol-Restricted Diet

The nutritional aim of a fructose- *plus* sorbitol-restricted diet is to limit the intake of foods rich in fructose and sorbitol to a level that does not trigger intestinal symptoms.

Table 31-2
Foods Containing Sorbitol and Other Sugar Alcohols

Fruits	*Dietetic Foods*	*Artificial Sweeteners*	*Others*
Apples	Jams	Sorbitol	Apple juice
Pears	Quince jelly	Mannitol	Pear juice
Apricots	Biscuits	Isomalt	Prune juice
Peaches	Ice cream	Xylitol	Sugar-free chewing gums
Plums	Chocolate		Sugar-free candies
Cherries			Sugar-free mints
Nectarines			Baked goods
Raisins			

As previously mentioned, the main determinants of fructose malabsorption from foods are the amount of fructose in excess of glucose and the intake of foods containing both fructose and sorbitol. I recommend that patients eliminate all foods with either excess free fructose or sorbitol from the diet (Tables 31-1 and 31-2).[6,22] Sucrose exclusion from the diet is unnecessary. Foods with an excess of free fructose may be better tolerated if glucose supplements are added to its consumption, with the aim of improving fructose absorption. In this sense, glucose-enriched sport drinks, glucose tablets or powder, glucose syrup, or glucose candies may be useful.

References

1. Rumessen JJ. Fructose and related food carbohydrates. Sources, intake, absorption, and clinical implications. *Scand J Gastroenterol.* 1992;27:819-828.
2. Caspary WF. Diarrhoea associated with carbohydrate malabsorption. *Clin Gastroenterol.* 1986;15:631-655.
3. Bleich SN, Wang YC, Wang Y, Gortmaker SL. Increasing consumption of sugar-sweetened beverages among US adults: 1988-1994 to 1999-2004. *Am J Clin Nutr.* 2009;89:372-381.
4. Vos MB, Kimmons JE. Dietary fructose consumption among US children and adults: the third National Health and Nutrition Examination Survey. *Medscape J Med.* 2008;10:160.
5. Park K, Yetley E. Intakes and food sources of fructose in the United States. *Am J Clin Nutr.* 1993;58 (suppl):737S-747S.
6. Fernández-Bañares F, Rosinach M, Esteve M, et al. Sugar malabsorption in functional abdominal bloating: a pilot study on the long-term effect of dietary treatment. *Clin Nutr.* 2006;25:824-831.
7. Nelis GF, Vermeeran MAP, Jansen W. Role of fructose-sorbitol mixtures in the symptoms of the irritable bowel. *Gastroenterology.* 1990;99:1016-1020.
8. Fernández Bañares F, Esteve-Pardo M, de Leon R, et al. Sugar malabsorption in functional bowel disease: clinical implications. *Am J Gastroenterol.* 1993;88:2044-2050.
9. Symons P, Jones MP, Kellow JE. Symptom provocation in irritable bowel syndrome. Effects of differing doses of fructose-sorbitol. *Scand J Gastroenterol.* 1992;27:940-944.
10. Gibson PR, Newnham E, Barrett JS, et al. Review article: fructose malabsorption and the bigger picture. *Aliment Pharmacol Ther.* 2007;25:349-363.
11. Ravich WJ, Bayless TM, Thomas M. Fructose: incomplete intestinal absorption in humans. *Gastroenterology.* 1983;84:26-29.

12. Fernández-Bañares F, Esteve M, Viver JM. Fructose-sorbitol malabsoption. *Curr Gastroenterol Rep.* 2009;11:368-374.
13. Simrén M, Stotzer PO. Use and abuse of hydrogen breath tests. *Gut.* 2006;55:297-303.
14. Vesa TH, Seppo LM, Marteau T, et al. Role of irritable bowel syndrome in subjective lactose intolerance. *Am J Clin Nutr.* 1998;67:710-715.
15. Goldstein R, Braverman D, Stankiewicz H. Carbohydrate malabsorption and the effect of dietary restriction on symptoms of irritable bowel syndrome and functional bowel complaints. *Isr Med Assoc J.* 2000;2:583-587.
16. Johlin FC, Panther M, Kraft N. Dietary fructose intolerance: diet modification can impact self-rated health and symptom control. *Nutr Clin Care.* 2004;7:92-94.
17. Choi YK, Kraft N, Zimmerman B, et al. Fructose intolerance in IBS and utility of fructose-restricted diet. *J Clin Gastroenterol.* 2008;42:233-238.
18. Born P, Sekatcheva M, Rösch T, Classen M. Carbohydrate malabsorption in clinical routine: a prospective observational study. *Hepatogastroenterology.* 2006;53:673-677.
19. Fernández-Bañares F, Esteve M, Salas A, et al. Systematic evaluation of the causes of chronic watery diarrhea with functional characteristics. *Am J Gastroenterol.* 2007;102:2520-2528.
20. Ledochowski M, Widner B, Bair H, et al. Fructose- and sorbitol-reduced diet improves mood and gastrointestinal disturbances in fructose malabsorbers. *Scand J Gastroenterol.* 2000;35:1048-1052.
21. Shepherd SJ, Parker FC, Muir JG, Gibson PR. Dietary triggers of abdominal symptoms in patients with irritable bowel syndrome: Randomized placebo-controlled evidence. *Clin Gastroenterol Hepatol.* 2008;6:765-771.
22. Barret JS, Gibson PR. Clinical ramifications of malabsorption of fructose and other short-chain carbohydrates. *Practical Gastroenterology.* 2007;31:51-65.

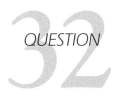
WHAT IS THE ROLE OF FIBER IN PATIENTS WITH IBS?

Anil Minocha, MD, FACP, FACG and Ankur Sheth, MD, MPH, FACP, CNSC

It is common practice to recommend a high-fiber diet or fiber supplements to irritable bowel syndrome (IBS) patients; however, there is conflicting evidence regarding the efficacy of this practice. Major limitations in previous studies that have evaluated the role of fiber in IBS patients include heterogeneous patient populations, a strong placebo effect, and nonstandardized outcome measures. In addition, most of the trials have been done in secondary or tertiary care settings, in spite of the fact that most patients with IBS are predominantly treated in primary care.

Types of Fiber

Fiber can be classified as soluble or insoluble based on its solubility in water. Soluble fibers are psyllium or ispaghula, partially hydrolyzed guar gum, and calcium polycarbophil. Insoluble fibers include wheat bran and corn bran. Fruits and vegetables contain substantial amounts of both soluble and insoluble fiber, while cereals, especially bran, contain mainly insoluble fiber.

Effect of Fiber in IBS

Ford and colleagues[1] recently published a meta-analysis of 12 trials comparing fiber with placebo or a low-fiber diet. Five studies used bran, six studies used ispaghula husk, and one used "concentrated" fiber of an unspecified type. Overall, 155 of 300 (52%) patients assigned to fiber had persistent or unimproved symptoms after treatment, compared to 168 of 291 (57%) allocated to placebo or a low-fiber diet (relative risk=0.87; 95% confidence interval 0.76 to 1.00, P=0.05). There was no statistically significant difference among the studies (I2=14.2%, P=0.31). The number needed to treat to prevent 1 patient with persistent symptoms was 11 (95% confidence interval 5 to 100). In a subgroup analysis, bran had no significant effect on IBS (relative risk of persistent or unimproved symptoms=1.02; 0.82

to 1.27). In contrast, ispaghula was effective in treating IBS (relative risk of persistent or unimproved symptoms=0.78; 0.63 to 0.96). The number needed to treat for ispaghula was 6 (3 to 50). No significant adverse effects were noted in the fiber group.

Effect of Soluble versus Insoluble Fiber

Soluble and insoluble fibers vary in their effects on IBS symptoms. Soluble fiber is more effective than insoluble fiber. A multicenter, randomized, open trial compared the effect of 30 g/day of wheat bran versus 5 g/day of partially hydrolyzed guar gum (PHGG). PHGG was associated with greater success (60% versus 40% in bran group) and was better tolerated and preferred by patients.[2]

Bijkerk and colleagues[3] in their meta-analysis compared the effects of soluble fiber (9 studies) and insoluble fiber (8 studies) separately on global and individual symptom relief from IBS. Fiber, in general, was effective in the relief of global IBS symptoms (relative risk=1.33; 95% confidence interval 1.19 to 1.50). Fiber provided benefit in constipation-predominant IBS (relative risk=1.56; 95% CI 1.21 to 2.02), but it did not relieve abdominal pain. Soluble fiber (psyllium, ispaghula, calcium polycarbophil) resulted in significant symptomatic improvement (relative risk=1.55; 95% CI 1.35 to 1.78). Insoluble fiber (corn, wheat bran), in some cases, worsened the clinical outcome; however, there was no significant difference compared to placebo (relative risk=0.89; 95% CI 0.72 to 1.11).

Use of Fiber in Primary- versus Secondary-Care Setting

Fiber seems to be more effective in the primary-care setting rather than secondary care, and this difference is likely because patients referred to specialists tend to have more severe symptoms and generally have already failed trials of fiber and/or fiber supplements. While most studies have been done in the secondary-care setting, Bijkerk and colleagues[4] evaluated the effect of 12 weeks of treatment with 10 g psyllium, 10 g bran, or 10 g placebo in IBS patients in a primary-care setting using a randomized, placebo-controlled fashion. At the end of the 3 months of treatment, symptom severity was reduced by 90 points in the psyllium group compared to 49 points among patients receiving placebo (P=0.03). In contrast, the score declined by only 58 points in the bran group (P=0.61).

Effect of Dose of Fiber

Only one study has attempted to define the optimal dose of a fiber supplement. Over 20 years ago, Kumar and colleagues[5] compared 20-, 30-, and 40-gram doses of ispaghula husk and concluded that the optimal dose of ispaghula husk in IBS is 20 g per day.

Effect of Fiber Intake in Food

Unlike fiber supplements, very few studies have examined the effect of increasing fiber intake in the form of ordinary food. In a single-blind, randomized, clinical trial, Aller and colleagues[6] studied 56 subjects who were randomly assigned to receive a diet containing 10.4 or 30.5 g/day of fiber. They reported improvement in IBS symptoms in patients taking both the high-fiber and low-fiber diets, a result they attributed to a placebo or Hawthorne effect.

American College of Gastroenterology Guidelines

In an evidence-based position statement on the management of IBS,[7] the American College of Gastroenterology IBS task force concluded that psyllium (ispaghula husk) is moderately effective. The same panel also concluded that wheat bran or corn bran is no more effective than placebo in the relief of global IBS symptoms and did not recommend its routine use.

Summary

- Fiber is effective in treating IBS-related symptoms, especially those of constipation. There is a high placebo response rate. Risk-benefit assessment suggests that fiber supplementation serves as a healthy, cheap, and effective placebo.

- Fiber supplementation is probably more effective in the primary-care setting than in the secondary-care setting.

- Soluble fiber should be the fiber of choice.

- Excessive intake of insoluble cereal fibers can worsen IBS symptoms, especially abdominal pain, in up to 50% of patients. Thus, it may be worthwhile to first recommend a trial of cereal fiber exclusion in some IBS patients, especially those with significant gas and bloating.

References

1. Ford AC, Talley NJ, Spiegel BM, et al. Effect of fibre, antispasmodics, and peppermint oil in the treatment of irritable bowel syndrome: systematic review and meta-analysis. *BMJ.* 2008;337:a2313.
2. Parisi GC, Zilli M, Miani MP, et al. High-fiber diet supplementation in patients with irritable bowel syndrome (IBS): a multicenter, randomized, open trial comparison between wheat bran diet and partially hydrolyzed guar gum (PHGG). *Dig Dis Sci.* 2002;47:1697-1704.
3. Bijkerk CJ, Muris JW, Knottnerus JA, Hoes AW, de Wit NJ. Systematic review: the role of different types of fibre in the treatment of irritable bowel syndrome. *Aliment Pharmacol Ther.* 2004;19:245-251.
4. Bijkerk CJ, de Wit NJ, Muris JW, Whorwell PJ, Knottnerus JA, Hoes AW. Soluble or insoluble fibre in irritable bowel syndrome in primary care? Randomised placebo controlled trial. *BMJ.* 2009;339:b3154.
5. Kumar A, Kumar N, Vij JC, Sarin SK, Anand BS. Optimum dosage of ispaghula husk in patients with irritable bowel syndrome: correlation of symptom relief with whole gut transit time and stool weight. *Gut.* 1987;28:150-155.
6. Aller R, de Luis DA, Izaola O, et al. Effects of a high-fiber diet on symptoms of irritable bowel syndrome: a randomized clinical trial. *Nutrition.* 2004;20:735-737.
7. Brandt LJ, Chey WD, Foxx-Orenstein AE, et al. An evidence-based position statement on the management of irritable bowel syndrome. *Am J Gastroenterol.* 2009;104(Suppl 1):S1-S35.

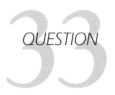
WHAT IS THE PLACEBO RESPONSE AND WHY IS IT SO HIGH IN PATIENTS WITH IBS?

W. Grant Thompson, MD, FRCPC

Have you pondered, as I do, the positive response of 20% to 40% of irritable bowel syndrome (IBS) subjects in the "placebo control group" of randomized controlled clinical trials? Or wondered how it was that blood-letting was commonly used over centuries to treat a host of mortal diseases, when a rationale is lacking and the dangers are obvious? Why do people patronize purveyors of alternative medicine who need not prove the efficacy nor define the dangers of their treatments? Why does a child with a scraped knee cease crying when comforted by his mom?

Faith, hope, and expectation are factors of course, but placebo responses are complex. This chapter discusses the elements that comprise the placebo response in general terms and concludes by urging their mobilization in the treatment of IBS. While placebo responses occur in most treatments, my discussion begins by illustrating the phenomenon with a treatment randomized controlled trial for a chronic painful condition, such as IBS or fibromyalgia (see box below and Figure 33-1).

Placebo response *is the response to placebo treatment in a clinical trial as illustrated by the second column in Figure 33-1. As explained in the caption, such a response is larger than the response to the treatment being tested. The principle determinants of the placebo response are the placebo effect and the benefit of time.*

Placebo effect *is the response to a treatment or placebo that is not due to treatment (drug) effect or the factors described next.*

(Continued on next page)

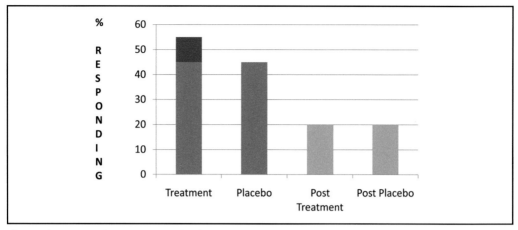

Figure 33-1. Result summary of a hypothetical randomized controlled trial comparing drug treatment to placebo for a chronic painful disorder such as IBS, headache, fibromyalgia, etc.

Note that about 55% of subjects typically respond to the drug treatment while only 45% respond to the placebo. The difference, in this case 10%, is known as the *therapeutic gain,* and such data are often sufficient to convince regulatory authorities to license a new drug.

Because this is a double-blind experiment and the treatment allocation is randomized, exactly the same conditions must prevail in both treatment and placebo groups. Thus, it is incorrect to say that the treatment response is 55%. Rather, in the treatment group, 45% of the improvement is due to the *placebo response* (same as that in the placebo group), and only 10% is due to the drug.

Whether or not 10% is sufficient to justify the drug's use is moot, but the point here is that the placebo response accounts for the greater share of the improvement. The principal components of the placebo response are *natural improvement* and the *placebo effect.*

Once the placebo or drug is withdrawn (light blue columns), some improvement remains (in this case 20%). In a natural experiment, this would indicate spontaneous improvement. However, this is a randomized controlled trial and, therefore, not natural. Factors such as *regression to the mean, parallel interventions,* and frequent monitoring must be considered, but the greatest healing determinant is the *placebo effect.*

Key: Red = therapeutic gain; dark blue = placebo response; light blue = placebo response after treatment withdrawal.

(Box continued)

Time effects *in a natural experiment would be the benefit of time and spontaneous improvement. However, in a randomized controlled trial, the circumstances are contrived, and other factors must also be considered:*

Regression to the mean. *Because, for trial purposes, patients currently suffering pain are selected from all those with the chronic, painful disorder, and because such disorders fluctuate in occurrence and intensity, some of the selected subjects will inevitably improve. If everyone with the diagnosis were entered in the trial (assuming this were possible), this skew phenomenon would not occur. Of course, there would be little point entering asymptomatic patients in a treatment randomized controlled trial.*

Parallel interventions *are those that accompany the administration of treatment and placebo in a randomized controlled trial. These include monitoring visits, explanations, and symptomatic interventions.*

Therapeutic Benefit = Treatment Effect + Placebo Response

The major healing determinants of the placebo response in a randomized controlled trial can be applied to all therapeutic encounters. Thus,

Placebo Response = Effects of time, regression to the mean, and parallel interventions + Placebo Effect

They must be deployed knowingly, compassionately, and without deceit.

Illness versus Disease

We must distinguish disease from illness. Disease is what a pathologist or physician can observe. It may be a peptic ulcer, seen as a crater in the lining of the stomach or duodenum, or diabetes, signified by a high blood-sugar test result. In such cases, the patient's symptoms have a tangible cause, and treatment can be logical and precise. In contrast, illness is what one feels. Illness may accompany a known disease, or not, but the patient feels ill. If the underlying disease is cured by appropriate treatment, the symptoms usually improve. However, what if there is illness without disease? Such illness is deemed due to a *functional disorder* and has no known cause.[1] Those suffering from such disorders will be disappointed to discover that there is no specific treatment. Nevertheless, despite the lack of a cure for functional disorders such as IBS, there are measures that you can deploy to alleviate the illness.

The Nature of Chronic Pain

Everyone experiences pain occasionally. Sometimes, the cause is obvious—pain from a clumsy hammer blow to the thumb or nausea from a rushed meal. Others have a medical explanation—abdominal pain due to a peptic ulcer or headache due to a neoplasm. Still others have no observable cause and are said to be functional. Pain and other symptoms with no conventional medical explanation are commonplace and begin in childhood. They include transient headaches, muscle pains, gut cramps, and numb extremities. We usually consider these to be inconsequential—part of living.

Symptoms such as pain are highly personal. Pain intrudes in our private world and is shared mainly through words. Facial grimaces and other nonverbal communication may let others know that we suffer, but they will not know from *what* we suffer until we tell them. We must struggle to understand the symptoms of a crying baby. We know when animals suffer, too, but they lack articulation so we cannot know the nature of their suffering. Although we may understand that another has pain, we must rely entirely on his or her words to discover its severity, location, and provoking factors. These are subject not only to the nature of the injury (if there is one), but also the prior experience, beliefs, and mood of the sufferer. We have no basis of comparison. We can judge with authority that our own pain is better, or worse, or the same, but we have no means of ranking it against that of other people.

Sometimes, symptoms become chronic, repetitive, and severe. There may be groups of symptoms that suggest a disturbance or *syndrome* in the intestines, the head, the bladder, the reproductive organs, or elsewhere. When these interfere with normal living or seem to warn of a disease, they prompt medical attention and become, at least for the moment, a medical problem. For some chronic functional disorders, no conventional medical explanation is available. IBS is a functional disorder whose defining characteristic is that the manifestly altered functioning of the gut's nerves, muscles, and hormones has no known cause.

Chronic pain of unknown origin is different from acute pain. The patient often has difficulty localizing the pain. IBS patients seldom use one finger to point to the affected area. The pain may move around, and local tenderness may be absent. It is often described without physical anguish and, because it fluctuates, may be absent at the time of examination. Sometimes, the symptom is described with extravagant language, such as "devastating" or "crippling," while the sufferer seems well and functioning and there are no physical findings. (If the pain becomes constant and disabling, it may be a chronic pain syndrome and is not further considered here.)

Placebo Effect in IBS

All treatments have the potential to elicit a placebo response, but no more than anecdotal evidence supports the notion that the placebo effect benefits disease. With terminal cancer treatments, there may be no structural benefit, but the placebo effect can lessen suffering. The placebo response is potentially greatest for the chronic, relapsing, and subjective pain of an illness such as IBS. Not only do the symptoms wax and wane, but diagnosis, reassurance, and empathy enhance the placebo effect.

The Therapeutic Relationship and Factors That Enhance the Placebo Effect

Many believe that medicine is a commodity and that treatments are standard and automatic. *Infection? Take a pill! Gall stones? Remove them!* Were that true, computers could replace doctors, and treatments could be auto-responses to typed-in complaints. But illness is too nuanced for binary computer programming, and every patient needs a careful human assessment. This interpersonal skill can neither be computerized nor delegated. Moreover, there is much more to healing than eliminating disease.

Disease is usually accompanied by illness—the discomfort, disability, suffering, and anxiety embraced by symptoms. Even with terminal disease, illness can be alleviated by compassion and by careful and collaborative deployment of the available treatment options. In functional disorders, there is no demonstrable disease, but often much illness. Bewilderment, embarrassment, fear, and other emotions aggravate the symptoms and impair a person's quality of life and functioning. You can help patients without specific treatment. There are no objective outcome measures here—no shrunken cancers or decreased fever—only the extent to which your patient feels better. This can best be achieved by wise exploitation of the placebo effect and of the known tendency of most functional symptoms, in most people, to improve from time to time.

What optimizes the placebo effect? Expectation and desire are important. If a patient expects you to help, then you are more likely to do so. Some improvement can be attributed to conditioning. If previous visits have had good outcomes, your patient may be conditioned to respond likewise this time.[2] (In an experiment, if a placebo is substituted *after* a course of an effective drug, it will be more effective than if it were given first.)

In another experiment, a pain-causing substance was injected into the skin of all four limbs of volunteers. Randomly, an inert cream was applied as treatment to some of the limbs. The volunteers expected the cream to relieve the pain in the treated limbs, and it did—but not those limbs to which no cream was applied. If you believe caffeine or alcohol will somehow improve your performance, they are more likely to do so than if you have doubts. Your patient's expectations of his or her consultation with you and its perceived realization can reinforce the benefits of treatment.

Much depends upon the therapeutic or doctor/patient relationship. It is said that the doctor is the placebo. Your reputation, profession, and demeanor build trust. The confidence, enthusiasm, and positivity with which you deliver care enhance your benefit to the patient. Even an office or clinic can create an atmosphere of healing—medicinal smells, diplomas, instruments, and bustling activity. The examination itself can be comforting. "At last, someone is taking my problem seriously!"

Diagnosis provides meaning for a patient. Only after diagnosis can you and your patient take the opportunity to discuss such things as prognosis, risks, and the nature of the illness. Only then can you provide the reassurance most patients with functional somatic complaints crave, particularly if they have consulted you because they feared serious disease.

When relief depends heavily upon your skill in alleviating a person's anxiety and fear, you become a healing instrument. You can inspire confidence, make a diagnosis, relieve anxiety, assuage fear, and express empathy. These objectives can be satisfied neither in a 5-minute visit nor by a computer with its background noise of misinformation and unsubstantiated cures. Because time costs money, and both are controlled by third parties, doctors and patients can do little to extend it. Yet, sufficient time is so important to the doctor-patient relationship that its provision should be just as much a part of the health-care effort as shorter wait times and technological availability. Lack of sufficient time for the therapeutic relationship has a *nocebo* effect.

Summary

There is no specific treatment proven to be effective for functional disorders. Even palliation through diet, lifestyle, antidiarrheals, laxatives, and psychoactive treatments are of marginal benefit in IBS. The strongest therapy is that provided by the therapeutic relationship. This should prompt you to make an early firm diagnosis, provide the expected diet and lifestyle advice, use the known data on the natural history of IBS to reassure the patient, and convince him or her that cancer is not the cause of the symptoms. Then, you should strive to mobilize the placebo effect through the ancient healing elements of empathy, explanation, reassurance, and a positive approach.

References

1. Thompson WG. *Understanding the Irritable Gut: The Functional Gastrointestinal Disorders.* McLean, VA: Degnon Press; 2008.
2. Thompson WG. *The placebo Effect and Health: Combining Science & Compassionate Care.* Amherst, NY: Prometheus Books; 2005.

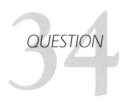

WHICH PATIENT WITH IBS IS LIKELY TO BENEFIT FROM SMOOTH MUSCLE ANTISPASMODICS?

Alexander Ford, MD

To answer this question, first one needs to be aware of the evidence for any benefit of antispasmodic drugs in irritable bowel syndrome (IBS), and, second, one has to take a pertinent history from the patient with whom one is consulting because of an exacerbation of their IBS symptoms. The majority of smooth muscle antispasmodic drugs, such as dycycloverine, hyoscine, and alverine, act chiefly by competing with acetylcholine at postganglionic parasympathetic nerve endings, thereby inhibiting smooth muscle contraction. Peppermint oil, which is a natural herbal remedy, also appears to have antispasmodic properties, but does not have the same mechanism of action and is thought to bring about smooth muscle relaxation via the blockade of calcium channels. Exactly how these pharmacological properties translate into a therapeutic effect in patients with IBS remains uncertain, but some researchers have shown, using magnetic resonance imaging, that diarrhea-predominant IBS patients have a reduced colon diameter, as well as accelerated small bowel transit. It may be that antispasmodics and peppermint oil act by reducing colonic contraction and decelerating intestinal transit time and, therefore, ameliorate the pain experienced by the patient, as well as decreasing their overall stool frequency.

A recent systematic review and meta-analysis of 22 randomized controlled trials of antispasmodic drugs and 4 trials of peppermint oil demonstrated that these agents are more effective than placebo in treating IBS.[1] The number needed to treat with antispasmodics to improve or cure one patient's symptoms was 5, while that for peppermint oil was 3. However, none of the included studies met the Rome committee's recommendations for the design of treatment trials in the functional gastrointestinal disorders,[2] and most of the trials failed to report either the method used to generate the randomization schedule or the method used to conceal allocation. The former limitation is unavoidable,

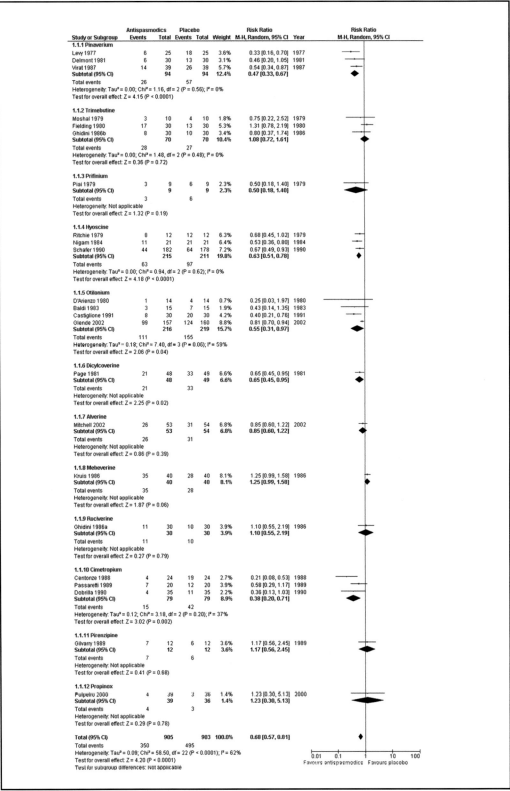

Figure 34-1. Forest plot of randomized controlled trials of antispasmotics versus placebo in irritable bowel syndrome.

as the majority of trials were designed and conducted before the guidelines from the Rome committee were published, while the latter shortcoming has been shown to lead to an overestimation of the benefit of the active drug under study. In addition, there were only limited data for many of the antispasmodics that are traditionally used in IBS, and the overall efficacy did not appear to be consistent across all the different drugs that were studied (Figure 34-1), suggesting that the observed benefit was not a true class-effect. There was only 1 trial using each of alverine, mebeverine, and dicycloverine, and of these only dicycloverine appeared to be of any benefit in IBS.

The best evidence, in terms of the number of trials and overall efficacy, appeared to exist for hyoscine, which was studied in 3 trials containing more than 400 patients, with a number needed to treat to prevent one patient's symptoms persisting of only 4. Unfortunately, this meta-analysis was unable to examine any benefit of different therapies according to the predominant stool pattern reported by the patient, because very few of the eligible trials reported these data, as the vast majority predated the widespread use of these IBS subgroups, making *post hoc* assignments of trial participants into these categories impossible. In terms of side effects, significantly more patients randomized to receive antispasmodics complained of adverse effects, compared with those receiving placebo, with a number needed to treat with antispasmodics to cause one adverse event of 18. The most common side effects reported were dry mouth, dizziness, and blurred vision. Adverse events with peppermint oil were fewer in number and did not occur significantly more often than with placebo.

A recent randomized controlled trial, published subsequent to this meta-analysis, has examined the efficacy of a combination of alverine and simethicone compared with placebo in IBS patients.[3] This reported that response rates were 47% with the alverine/simethicone combination versus 34% with placebo. Unfortunately, once again, the effect of active therapy according to predominant stool pattern was not reported in the published trial, despite the fact that it was designed and conducted subsequent to the widespread use of these subgroups. If one assumes that alverine is the only active component in the alverine/simethicone combination, and these data are incorporated into the aforementioned meta-analysis, then alverine is also more effective than placebo in the treatment of IBS, with a number needed to treat of 8, in 2 trials containing more than 500 patients.

With this knowledge in mind, I try to elicit from the patient his or her predominant symptom. Given the pharmacological properties of smooth muscle antispasmodics and peppermint oil discussed above, it would seem reasonable to assume that these agents are likely to be most beneficial in IBS patients who have diarrhea as their predominant stool pattern and/or who report pain as a major feature during exacerbations of their disease activity. If diarrhea, combined with pain, is present and this is the predominant symptom reported by the patient, I will give the patient a trial of peppermint oil, at a dose of 2 capsules 3 times daily, due to the low side effect profile. Where this fails, I use hyoscine at a dose of 10 mg 3 times daily, increasing to 20 mg 3 times daily if there is no response initially, warning the patient about the potential side effects. If hyoscine is of no benefit, then a trial of another antispasmodic drug is probably worthwhile before escalating therapy, and, in the light of recent evidence, it would seem reasonable to try alverine in this situation.

References

1. Ford AC, Talley NJ, Spiegel BMR, et al. Efficacy of fibre, antispasmodics, and peppermint oil in irritable bowel syndrome: Systematic review and meta-analysis. *Br Med J.* 2008;337:1388-1392.
2. Design of Treatment Trials Committee, Irvine EJ, Whitehead WE, Chey WD, et al. Design of treatment trials for functional gastrointestinal disorders. *Gastroenterology.* 2006;130:1538-1551.
3. Wittmann T, Paradowski L, Ducrotte P, Bueno L, Andro Delestrain MC. Clinical trial: efficacy of alverine citrate/simeticone combination on abdominal pain/discomfort in irritable bowel syndrome: results of a randomized, double-blind, placebo-controlled study. *Aliment Pharmacol Ther.* 2010;31:615-624.

Note: Although available and widely used in Canada and Europe, dycycloverine, mebeverine, hyoscine, and alverine are not currently available in the United States.

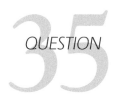

WHAT IS THE ROLE OF TRICYCLIC ANTIDEPRESSANTS IN THE TREATMENT OF IBS?

Paul Moayyedi, BSc, MB, ChB, PhD, MPH, FRCP, FRCPC, AGAF, FACG

Tricyclic antidepressants (TCAs), like the early antipsychotics, were developed from antihistamines with the aim to sedate disturbed psychiatric patients. They were first synthesized in the 1950s and derive their name from the three-amine ring structure that is common to this class of drugs. They have a variety of pharmacological actions, including serotonin and norepinephrine-reuptake inhibition as well as muscarinic, histaminic, and α_1 adrenergic blockade.[1] TCAs have been shown to improve depressive symptoms in randomized controlled trials (RCTs), but the precise mechanisms by which they achieve this are unclear, which perhaps is not surprising given the diverse pharmacological actions of these drugs.

Depressed patients often have chronic pain syndromes, and it was noted that pain symptoms were also improved by TCAs. This observation was confirmed by several RCTs. A Cochrane systematic review[2] identified 17 RCTs involving 724 patients that evaluated the efficacy of TCAs in neuropathic pain and found these drugs were effective with a number needed to treat (NNT) of 4 (95% confidence interval [CI] 3 to 5) to produce at least a moderate improvement in pain compared to placebo.

The Evidence for TCAs in IBS

The cardinal symptom of irritable bowel syndrome (IBS) is abdominal pain so it is plausible that TCAs will also be beneficial for this disorder. Initial RCTs were not promising, and an early Cochrane systematic review[3] suggested there was no clear evidence that TCAs were beneficial in IBS. Since then, however, there have been a number of RCTs and a further systematic review,[4] and it has become clear that TCAs do have

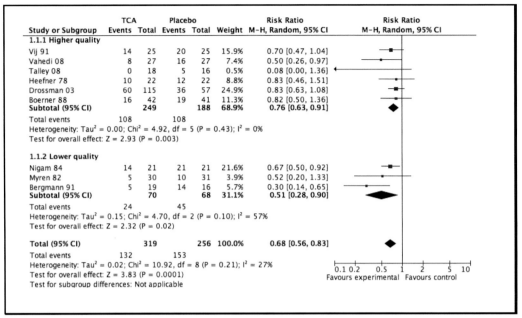

Figure 35-1. Forest plot of RCTs evaluating TCAs versus placebo in IBS patients. Relative risk of IBS symptoms remains unchanged.

a role in IBS, as in other chronic pain syndromes. The systematic review reported on nine trials that evaluated 575 IBS patients.[4] A variety of TCAs were utilized including amitriptyline, doxepin, trimipramine, imipramine, and desipramine, and patients were followed for 4 to 12 weeks. Only three studies showed a statistically significant reduction in global symptoms in those randomized to TCA versus placebo but all reported a trend toward TCAs benefiting IBS symptoms. When data were pooled in the systematic review,[4] there was a clear benefit of active treatment with a NNT of 4 (95% CI 3 to 6). This effect is probably overestimated as the higher quality studies showed less variation in outcome and overall had a lower treatment effect with an NNT of 6 (95% CI 4 to 12.5) (Figure 35-1).

The mechanism of action of these drugs is unclear. Patients with IBS are more likely to have depression, so it is possible that TCAs are acting by simply improving mood. This hypothesis has not been addressed adequately in trials, although three studies have reported that any impact on IBS symptoms seemed to be independent of any effect on depression. Indeed, many trials used low doses of TCAs, and so any effect of these drugs on mood is likely to be limited. The lack of correlation between TCA efficacy on pain and effect on mood has also been noted in chronic pain trials.[2] The authors of these trials reported that patients respond after a few days, long before these drugs should have any effect on depression. Trials have also suggested the TCAs are effective in patients with chronic pain who are not depressed. It is likely, therefore, that TCAs act by either altering the central processing of pain or having a peripheral neuromodulating role.

Role of TCAs in IBS

There is no "magic bullet" to treat IBS, and all therapeutic options have their advantages and disadvantages. The evidence that TCAs are effective in IBS is persuasive, although it would be reassuring to have more RCT data and a better understanding of the mechanism of action. These drugs have been used for a long time and are relatively inexpensive but have significant side effects. Adverse events are particularly related to the anticholinergic effects of TCAs and include drowsiness, blurred vision, urinary retention, and constipation. TCAs are also associated with arrhythmias, tachycardia, palpitations, and heart block and should be used with caution in those with significant heart disease. TCAs appear to be effective at very low doses, while the adverse effects of these drugs increase with increasing dosage. It, therefore, makes sense to use these drugs at the lowest available dose (eg, 10 or 12.5 mg for amitriptyline) to minimize any risk.

Guidelines[5] recommend that TCAs are used second line in IBS patients after first-line therapies, such as fiber and antispasmodics, have failed. They may be particularly useful when pain is the predominant problem. Because these drugs can cause constipation, they may not be ideal for constipation-predominant IBS and are probably better suited for those with diarrhea-predominant or alternating IBS patients. This recommendation, however, is not evidence based, and trials have not looked at this question specifically. Drowsiness can be an issue, and so patients may prefer to take their medication before bedtime.

Summary

TCAs have an important role in IBS, particularly when pain is a major issue for patients. There is reasonable randomized trial evidence that these drugs are effective, and at low doses, they are usually well tolerated. Caution should be used in the elderly and those with multiple comorbidities, particularly those with heart disease. Nevertheless, they are a useful treatment option in what is a difficult disorder to treat.

References

1. Godfrey RG. A guide to the understanding and use of tricyclic antidepressants in the overall management of fibromyalgia and other chronic pain syndromes. *Arch Intern Med.* 1996;156:1047-1052.
2. Saarto T, Wiffen PJ. Antidepressants for neuropathic pain. *Cochrane Database of Systematic Reviews.* 2007;Issue 4, Art. No.: CD005454. DOI: 10.1002/14651858.CD005454.pub2.
3. Quartero AO, Meiniche-Schmidt V, Muris J, Rubin G, de Wit N. Bulking agents, antispasmodic and antidepressant medication for the treatment of irritable bowel syndrome. *Cochrane Database of Systematic Reviews.* 2005;Issue 2, Art. No.: CD003460. DOI: 10.1002/14651858.CD003460.pub2.
4. Ford AC, Talley NJ, Schoenfeld PS, Quigley EMM, Moayyedi P. Efficacy of antidepressants and psychological therapies in irritable bowel syndrome: systematic review and meta-analysis. *Gut.* 2009;58:367-378.
5. Brandt LJ, Chey WD, Foxx-Orenstein AE, et al. An evidence-based systematic review on the management of irritable bowel syndrome: American College of Gastroenterology Task Force on IBS. *Am J Gastroenterol.* 2009;104(Suppl 1):S1-S35.

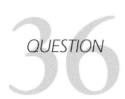

WHAT IS THE ROLE OF SSRIS IN THE TREATMENT OF IBS?

Jan Tack, MD, PhD

Irritable bowel syndrome (IBS) is probably the most commonly encountered disorder by gastroenterologists in the industrialized world. It is defined by the presence of abdominal pain associated with altered bowel habits, in the absence of organic disease.[1] For patients requiring pharmacotherapy, a number of first-line therapies, which mainly target stool pattern or colonic contractions, are often used in IBS.[2]

Traditionally, tricyclic antidepressants have been used to treat IBS patients, who fail to respond to reassurance and first-line therapies.[2-5] Initially, the rationale for their use was the high prevalence of comorbid depression and anxiety disorders in IBS patients.[6,7] However, the doses used are well below the doses used for depression or anxiety, and tricyclic agents also have neuromodulatory and analgesic properties. In addition, tricyclic agents have a number of different pharmacological actions including serotonin reuptake inhibition and anticholinergic actions. A number of studies have confirmed the efficacy of low-dose tricyclic antidepressants in IBS,[4,8,9] but it remains unclear whether the therapeutic efficacy of tricyclic agents in IBS is through their action on mood or anxiety, through central or peripheral neuromodulatory effects, or through analgesic actions. More recently, the crucial role of serotonin in the physiology of the gastrointestinal tract is increasingly being appreciated,[10] and it is now clear that serotonin reuptake inhibition may have profound effects on the control of gastrointestinal sensorimotor function.

Influence of Serotonin Reuptake Inhibitors on Intestinal Sensorimotor Function

Serotonin (5-HT) is a key neuromodulator and neurotransmitter in the control of gastrointestinal sensorimotor function.[10] In response to the presence of a bolus in the lumen of the gastrointestinal tract, enterochromaffin cells release 5-HT, which triggers peristaltic and secretory reflexes through the activation of intrinsic and extrinsic neural pathways. Serotonin is also involved in afferent signaling from the gastrointestinal tract to the brain.[10] The action of 5-HT is terminated when it is removed from the intercellular space by the serotonin transporter (SERT), which is expressed by enterocytes and nerves in the gastrointestinal tract.[10-13] Acute administration of selective serotonin reuptake inhibitors (SSRIs) prolongs the availability of physiologically released serotonin, thereby enhancing the effects of serotonin released from the gastrointestinal tract but also from the central nervous system.

To investigate whether inhibition of SERT function would alter colonic sensorimotor function in man, we used an SSRI to study the effect of SERT inhibition in a colonic barostat and manometry study.[11,14,15] Because longer-term use of SSRIs eventually leads to receptor desensitization,[16] we focused on the effects of acute intravenous administration. In healthy volunteers, acute intravenous administration of citalopram increased colonic phasic contractility and increased the frequency of occurrence of high-amplitude propagated contractions. At the same time, citalopram increased colonic compliance and suppressed the colonic tonic response to a meal.[15] These findings suggest involvement of 5-HT in both phasic contractility and tone of the human colon. Stimulation of colonic contractility could potentially benefit IBS patients with constipation. A reduction in colonic tone and suppression of meal-induced tonic response could decrease colonic sensitivity to volume distension and could inhibit meal-related increases in IBS symptom severity.[15,17]

The effects of SSRIs on small bowel motility were also studied. In the small bowel, short-term (5 days) oral pretreatment with paroxetine increased the occurrence of phase III of the migrating motor complex (MMC).[18,19] The effects of SSRIs and TCAs on small bowel and whole gut transit were studied in healthy controls and in a small group of patients with IBS.[20] Whereas SSRIs reduced orocecal transit times without a significant effect on whole gut transit times, TCAs prolonged orocecal transit and whole gut transit times, probably because of the anticholinergic profile on the latter.[20] Stimulation of small bowel motility by SSRIs could potentially be beneficial in IBS patients with constipation, but could be undesirable in IBS with diarrhea.

Efficacy of SSRIs in IBS Management

Seven relatively small placebo-controlled studies of SSRIs in IBS have been published, of which 4 reported symptomatic benefit of the SSRI over placebo.[21-27] These are summarized in Table 36-1. A meta-analysis of the first 5 studies, in which a total of 230 patients were studied, found an overall significant benefit with a relative risk of IBS symptoms persisting during SSRI therapy compared to placebo of 0.62 (95% CI, 0.45 to 0.87) and a number needed to treat of 3.5.[9] Since then, a sixth study, in which 54 patients were randomized to citalopram or placebo, however, also failed to show significant benefit[26] while a seventh study of paroxetine in 72 IBS patients was positive on a number of endpoints, but not the primary endpoint of a composite pain score.[27] Overall, these findings point toward absence of a major general beneficial effect, but likely benefit in a subset of patients. Symptoms that were reported to respond to SSRIs included abdominal pain or discomfort and bloating according to 2 studies,[23,24] while other studies were more suggestive of beneficial effects on general well-being.[22,27] The onset of therapeutic benefit seems to occur relatively rapidly, within the first 3 to 4 weeks.

Table 36-1

SSRIs in the Treatment of IBS

Study (Reference)	Number of Patients	Agents	Duration	Result
Kuiken et al[21]	40	• Fluoxetine 20 mg/day or • Placebo	6 weeks, parallel design	No significant benefit
Tabas et al[22]	90	• Paroxetine, 10, 20 to 40 mg or • Placebo	12 weeks	Improvement of overall well-being
Vahedi et al[23]	44	• Fluoxetine 20 mg or • Placebo	12 weeks	Improvement of abdominal discomfort, sense of bloating; increased frequency of bowel movements and decreased stool consistency
Tack et al[24]	23	• Citalopram 20 mg for 3 weeks and then 40 mg or • Placebo	6 weeks, cross-over design	Improvement of abdominal pain, bloating, impact of symptoms on daily life, and overall well-being
Talley et al[25]	51	• Imipramine 50 mg or • Citalopram 40 mg or • Placebo	12 weeks	No significant benefit
Ladabaum et al[26]	54	• Citalopram 20 mg for 4 weeks and then 40 mg or • Placebo	8 weeks	No significant benefit
Masand et al[27]	72	• Paroxetine CR 12.5 to 50 mg or • Placebo	12 weeks	No difference in composite pain scores; significantly higher response on Clinical Global Impression-Improvement

The mechanism underlying the beneficial effect of SSRIs remains unclear. Stimulation of small intestinal motility and transit could be beneficial to IBS patients with constipation. However, only one study focused on IBS with constipation[21]; the others included IBS patients regardless of their dominant stool pattern, and stool pattern did not seem to determine efficacy. It is conceivable that SSRIs might be beneficial through their effects on coexisting major anxiety and depression. However, most studies excluded patients with major anxiety or depression, and the therapeutic effect of SSRIs in the positive studies seemed unrelated to effects on anxiety or depression.[21-26,28] SSRIs also have some analgesic properties, given their application in neuropathic pain conditions. An effect on visceral hypersensitivity could be beneficial in IBS, but in several studies, SSRIs did not significantly alter rectal or colonic sensitivity.[21,24,26] Hence, the mechanism underlying potentially beneficial effects of SSRIs remains to be determined.

In contrast to the TCA studies, studies in IBS used the SSRIs at the usual antidepressant doses, with treatment durations between 6 and 12 weeks. In all studies, SSRIs were well tolerated, and withdrawals due to adverse events have been rare.

Implications for Clinical Management

As efficacy of SSRIs was found in only a subset of studies, they cannot be considered a first-line therapy for the treatment of IBS. In keeping with guidelines, SSRIs can be considered when first-line therapies, which mainly target stool pattern or colonic contractions, have failed to provide a response.

Although this has not been addressed specifically in the trials, it seems logical that a beneficial effect can be expected in IBS patients with clinically overt coexisting anxiety or depression. Compared to TCAs, the SSRIs have the advantage of not inducing constipation and of a good tolerance profile, which allows clinicians to use the higher doses used in the treatment of depression. Evidently, anti-depressive effects may take longer than the effects on IBS symptoms, which seem to occur after 3 to 4 weeks.

In patients without relevant anxiety or depression comorbidity, SSRIs can also be applied. They are an attractive alternative in the patient refractory to first- and second-line therapies (such as lubiprostone and, in the near future perhaps, linaclotide). SSRIs are especially attractive for use in IBS patients without diarrhea, as they do not induce or worsen constipation. Studies with SSRIs have used citalopram, paroxetine, and fluoxetine. At this time, there is no evidence for any of these to be superior to another, but it has been suggested that paroxetine may also have some anticholinergic properties.[29]

The best dose to use is probably the standard antidepressive dose, as this has been most widely studied. Given their stimulatory effects, many clinicians will avoid SSRIs in IBS with diarrhea, although the available studies usually did not exclude this group of patients. Explanation of the key role of 5-HT in gastrointestinal sensorimotor function and of the effects of SSRIs on gastrointestinal 5-HT function may help to enhance patient compliance with a drug that is primarily, as is written in the patient information, viewed as an antidepressant. In addition, similar to what is observed in depression, transient nausea may occur in the initial days of treatment. Evaluation of the therapeutic response can be done after 6 to 8 weeks of therapy. In case of insufficient response, doubling the dose could be considered, as some studies evaluated higher doses of SSRIs in IBS.[24,26]

Research Agenda

At present, a well-designed, large, multicenter study with an SSRI in IBS is lacking, and this would be needed to fully establish the presence of therapeutic efficacy and its magnitude. Although increasingly used clinically, no data are available on the efficacy of a class of related compounds, the serotonin/noradrenaline reuptake inhibitors, in IBS. Finally, the use of a peripherally selective serotonin reuptake inhibitor is an attractive concept, both from a pathophysiological and a therapeutic point of view. Such drugs are presently not available.

References

1. Longstreth GF, Thompson WG, Chey WD, Houghton LA, Mearin F, Spiller RC. Functional bowel disorders. *Gastroenterology.* 2006;130(5):1480-1491.
2. Tack J, Fried M, Houghton LA, Spicak J, Fisher G. Systematic review: the efficacy of treatments for irritable bowel syndrome—a European perspective. *Aliment Pharmacol Ther.* 2006;24(2):183-205.
3. Talley NJ. Antidepressants in IBS: are we deluding ourselves? *Am J Gastroenterol.* 2004;99:921-923.
4. Drossman DA, Toner BB, Whitehead WE, et al. Cognitive-behavioral therapy versus education and desipramine versus placebo for moderate to severe functional bowel disorders. *Gastroenterology.* 2003; 125(1):19-31.
5. Mertz HR. Irritable bowel syndrome. *N Engl J Med.* 2003;349:2136-2146.
6. Henningsen P, Zimmermann T, Sattel H. Medically unexplained physical symptoms, anxiety and depression: a meta-analytic review. *Psychosom Med.* 2003;65:528-533.
7. Sykes MA, Blanchard EB, Lackner J, et al. Psychopathology in irritable bowel syndrome: support for a psychophysiological model. *J Behav Med.* 2003;26:361-372.
8. Jackson JL, O'Malley PG, Tomkins G, Balden E, Santoro J, Kroenke K. Treatment of functional gastrointestinal disorders with antidepressant medications: a meta-analysis. *Am J Med.* 2000;108:65-72.
9. Ford AC, Talley NJ, Schoenfeld PS, et al. Efficacy of antidepressants and psychological therapies in irritable bowel syndrome: systematic review and meta-analysis. *Gut.* 2009;58:367-378.
10. Gershon M, Tack J. The serotonin signaling system: from basic understanding to drug development for functional GI disorders. *Gastroenterology.* 2007;132:397-414.
11. Gershon M, Jonakait G. Uptake and release of 5-hydroxytryptamine by enteric 5-hydroxytryptaminergic neurones: effects of fluoxetine and chlorimipramine. *Br J Pharmacol.* 1979;66:7-9.
12. Wade PR, Chen J, Jaffe B, Kassem IS, Blakely RD, Gershon MD. Localization and function of a 5-HT transporter in crypt epithelia of the gastrointestinal tract. *J Neurosci.* 1996;16:2352-2364.
13. Chen JX, Pan H, Rothman TP, Wade PR, Gershon MD. Guinea pig 5-HT transporter: cloning, expression, distribution, and function in intestinal sensory reception. *Am J Physiol.* 1998;275:G433-G448.
14. Qian Y, Melikian HE, Rye DB, Levey AI, Blakely RD. Identification and characterization of antidepressant-sensitive serotonin transporter proteins using site-specific antibodies. *J Neurosci.* 1995;15:1261-1274.
15. Tack J, Broekaert D, Corsetti M, Fischler B, Janssens J. Influence of acute serotonin reuptake inhibition on colonic sensorimotor function in man. *Aliment Pharmacol Ther.* 2006;23(2):265-274.
16. Bonhomme N, Esposito E. Involvement of serotonin and dopamine in the mechanism of action of novel antidepressant drugs: a review. *J Clin Psychopharmacol.* 1998;18(6):447-454.
17. Ragnarsson G, Bodemar G. Pain is temporally related to eating but not to defaecation in the irritable bowel syndrome (IBS). Patients' description of diarrhea, constipation and symptom variation during a prospective 6-week study. *Eur J Gastroenterol Hepatol.* 1998;10(5):415-421.
18. Chial HJ, Camilleri M, Burton D, Thomforde G, Olden KW, Stephens D. Selective effects of serotonergic psychoactive agents on gastrointestinal functions in health. *Am J Physiol Gastrointest Liver Physiol.* 2003; 284(1):G130-G137.
19. Gorard DA, Libby GW, Farthing MJG. 5-Hydroxytryptamine and human small intestinal motility: effect of inhibiting 5-hydroxytryptamine reuptake. *Gut.* 1994;35:496-500.
20. Gorard DA, Libby GW, Farthing MJ. Influence of antidepressants on whole gut and orocaecal transit times in health and irritable bowel syndrome. *Aliment Pharmacol Ther.* 1994;8(2):159-166.
21. Kuiken SD, Tytgat GN, Boeckxstaens GE. The selective serotonin reuptake inhibitor fluoxetine does not change rectal sensitivity and symptoms in patients with irritable bowel syndrome: a double blind, randomized, placebo-controlled study. *Clin Gastroenterol Hepatol.* 2003;1(3):219-228.
22. Tabas G, Beaves M, Wang J, Friday P, Mardini H, Arnold G. Paroxetine to treat irritable bowel syndrome not responding to high-fiber diet: a double-blind, placebo-controlled trial. *Am J Gastroenterol.* 2004;99(5): 914-920.
23. Vahedi H, Merat S, Rashidioon A, Ghoddoosi A, Malekzadeh R. The effect of fluoxetine in patients with pain and constipation-predominant irritable bowel syndrome: a double-blind randomized-controlled study. *Aliment Pharmacol Ther.* 2005;22(5):381-385.
24. Tack J, Broekaert D, Fischler B, Oudenhove LV, Gevers AM, Janssens J. A controlled crossover study of the selective serotonin reuptake inhibitor citalopram in irritable bowel syndrome. *Gut.* 2006;55(8):1095-1103.

25. Talley NJ, Kellow JE, Boyce P, et al. Antidepressant therapy (imipramine and citalopram) for irritable bowel syndrome: a double-blind, randomized, placebo controlled trial. *Dig Dis Sci.* 2008;53:108-115.

26. Ladabaum U, Sharabidze A, Levin TR, et al. Citalopram provides little or no benefit in nondepressed patients with irritable bowel syndrome. *Clin Gastroenterol Hepatol.* 2010;8(1):42-48.e1.

27. Masand PS, Pae CU, Krulewicz S, et al. A double-blind, randomized, placebo-controlled trial of paroxetine controlled-release in irritable bowel syndrome. *Psychosomatics.* 2009;50(1):78-86.

28. Marks DM, Han C, Krulewicz S, et al. History of depressive and anxiety disorders and paroxetine response in patients with irritable bowel syndrome: post hoc analysis from a placebo-controlled study. *Prim Care Companion J Clin Psychiatry.* 2008;10(5):368-375.

29. Stahl S. *Essential Psychopharmacology: Neuroscientific Basis and Practical Applications.* 2nd ed. Cambridge, UK: Cambridge University Press; 2000.

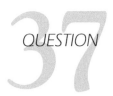
WHAT IS THE ROLE OF RIFAXIMIN IN THE TREATMENT OF IBS?

Philip Schoenfeld, MD, MSEd, MSc (Epi)

Rifaximin is a broad-spectrum antibiotic that has antimicrobial activity against many organisms in the gastrointestinal (GI) tract, including gram-negative rods and anaerobes. It is also unique because less than 0.4% of rifaximin is absorbed when taken orally. Because many antibiotic-associated side effects occur after absorption and are systemic in nature, the side effect profile of rifaximin should be minimal. Most importantly, 5 appropriately designed, placebo-controlled, randomized controlled trials (RCTs)[1-5] in more than 2000 IBS patients demonstrate that rifaximin-treated patients experience more relief of global IBS symptoms, bloating, and abdominal pain than placebo-treated IBS patients. Based on these RCT data, the ideal patient population for rifaximin is the nonconstipation-predominant IBS patient, especially those IBS patients who complain of bloating. The most appropriate dosage is 550 mg orally 3 times daily for 14 days. Based on available data,[5,6] patients with a positive response to rifaximin may expect IBS symptom relief for 3 to 6 months, and some patients may experience symptom relief for longer than 6 months. Long-term management of IBS patients with rifaximin has not been defined, although a small retrospective study[7] suggests that IBS patients respond well to a repeat course of rifaximin if/when their IBS symptoms relapse.

The Phase II[1,2] and Phase III[5] RCTs were well designed, meeting all criteria for appropriately designed RCTs (ie, truly randomized studies with concealment of treatment allocation, implementation of masking, completeness of follow-up, and intention-to-treat analysis). As well, these studies met most criteria suggested by the Rome committee for the design of treatment trials of functional GI disorders (eg, patients met Rome criteria for IBS, no placebo run-in, baseline observation of patients to assess IBS symptoms, and the primary study outcome is the improvement in global IBS symptoms). The other two RCTs[3,4] also met most criteria for appropriately designed RCTs. These RCTs demonstrated that rifaximin-treated patients were 8% to 23% more likely to experience global improvement in IBS symptoms, bloating symptoms, or abdominal pain compared with placebo-treated patients.

In the Phase II RCTs,[1,2] 388 diarrhea-predominant IBS patients were randomized to rifaximin 550 mg twice daily for 14 days followed by placebo for another 2 weeks, or, alternatively, they took placebo for 4 weeks. In this trial, patients had to experience adequate relief of IBS symptoms in 2 of 3 weeks to be considered a responder. Rifaximin-treated patients were significantly more likely to be responders compared to those treated with placebo (52.4 versus 44.2%, $P=0.03$). Notably, most of the improvement was not noted until 1 week after completion of the course of treatment.

Based on data from the Phase II RCT, the Phase III RCT[5] enrolled diarrhea-predominant IBS patients as well as mixed-IBS patients (ie, IBS patients with components of diarrhea, constipation, and normal stool consistency/frequency). Only IBS patients with constipation-predominant IBS were excluded. Study patients also demonstrated mild-moderate bloating during the 2-week run-in period prior to randomization to rifaximin or placebo. With these data, it appears that nonconstipated IBS patients with mild-moderate bloating may be ideal for rifaximin treatment. In the Phase III RCT, patients were randomized to rifaximin 550 mg three times daily for 14 days or placebo for 14 days. Patients were then observed for 10 weeks after completion of study treatment. Patients had to experience relief of IBS symptoms for 2 of 4 weeks after completion of study treatment to be considered a responder. Rifaximin-treated patients were more likely than placebo-treated patients to be responders for global IBS symptom relief (40.7% versus 31.7%, $P<0.001$), bloating (40.2% versus 30.3%, $P<0.001$), and daily assessment of abdominal pain (43.6% versus 35.3%, $P<0.001$). This improvement in responders was maintained for the duration of the 10-week study follow-up period.

Safety data from the Phase III RCTs is particularly promising. No difference in side effects was observed between rifaximin-treated patients and placebo-treated patients for any side effect, including headache (4.0% versus 4.4%), abdominal pain (2.7% versus 2.7%), nausea (2.6% versus 1.9%), or upper respiratory tract infection (0.6% versus 2.2%).

The mechanism of symptom relief for rifaximin in IBS patients is unclear, although experts hypothesize that rifaximin alters gut bacterial flora that resolves small intestinal bacterial overgrowth. Studies have also demonstrated that some IBS patients have increased levels of unstable mast cells in colonic mucosa and increased levels of lymphocytes around the myenteric plexus. This could lead to inflammation in the colonic mucosa, and experts also hypothesize that rifaximin resolves inflammation and normalizes immune system function in colonic mucosa, possibly by modifying gut bacterial flora.

Although the initial RCTs only enrolled IBS patients with small intestinal bacterial overgrowth based upon positive hydrogen or glucose breath testing, Phase II and Phase III RCTs of rifaximin did not perform breath testing on study patients. Therefore, it is not required to obtain positive breath tests before treating IBS patients with rifaximin, although current treatment should be limited to nonconstipation-predominant IBS patients.

The reader should note that rifaximin is not currently approved by the FDA for the treatment of IBS. Currently, rifaximin is approved by the FDA for treatment of traveler's diarrhea (200 mg orally twice daily for 3 days) and hepatic encephalopathy (550 mg orally twice daily). The dose of rifaximin used in the Phase III RCTs was 550 mg orally three times daily, and this dosage is efficacious based on the RCT data. Because the Phase III RCTs provide the most robust data, this is probably the most appropriate dose to use in an IBS patient.

Other antibiotics have been studied for treatment of IBS. With the exception of a small RCT of neomycin, no other antibiotic has demonstrated efficacy in the treatment of IBS.

References

1. Ringel Y, Palsson OS, Zakko SF, et al. Predictors of clinical response from a phase 2 multi-center efficacy trial using rifaximin, a gut-selective, nonabsorbed antibiotic for the treatment of diarrhea associated irritable bowel syndrome. *Gastroenterology.* 2008;134(Suppl 1):A550 (T1141).
2. Lembo A, Zakko SF, Ferreira NL, et al. Rifaximin for the treatment of diarrhea associated irritable bowel syndrome: short term treatment leading to long term sustained response. *Gastroenterology.* 2008;134(Suppl 1): A545 (T1390).
3. Sharara AI, Aoun E, Abdul-Baki H, et al. A randomized double-blind placebo-controlled trial of rifaximin in patients with abdominal bloating and flatulence. *Am J Gastroenterol.* 2006;101:326-333.
4. Pimentel M, Park S, Mirocha J, et al. The effect of a nonabsorbed oral antibiotic (rifaximin) on the symptoms of the irritable bowel syndrome: a randomized trial. *Ann Intern Med.* 2006;145:557-663.
5. Pimentel M, Lembo A, Chey WD, et al. Rifaximin therapy for patients with irritable bowel syndrome without constipation. *N Engl J Med.* 2011;364:22-32.
6. Lauritano EC, Gabrielli M, Scarpellini E, et al. Small intestinal bacterial overgrowth recurrence after antibiotic therapy. *Am J Gastroenterol.* 2008;103:2031-2035.
7. Yang J, Lee HR, Low K, et al. Rifaximin versus other antibiotics in the primary treatment and retreatment of bacterial overgrowth in IBS. *Dig Dis Sci.* 2008;53:169-174.

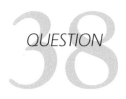

WHAT IS LUBIPROSTONE AND WHEN SHOULD I USE IT IN MY PATIENTS WITH IBS?

Lucinda A. Harris, MD and Tisha N. Lunsford, MD

Lubiprostone (Amitiza [Sucampo Pharmaceuticals, Inc, Bethesda, MD]) is a bicyclic fatty acid that is a member of a new class of agents called prostones. It was approved for the treatment of chronic idiopathic constipation (CIC) in *both* men and women in 2006 at a dose of 24 µg twice daily, and it was approved in 2008 at a dose of 8 µg twice daily for the treatment of **women** with irritable bowel syndrome with constipation (IBS-C).[1,2]

Using a new therapy requires an understanding of the drug's mechanism of action and metabolism. Lubiprostone is a type-2 chloride channel activator, and currently nine types of chloride channels are known to exist in humans.[3] The most recognized chloride channel is the cystic fibrosis transmembrane conductance regulator (CFTR), which is located on the intestinal epithelium. This channel is responsible for handling a major portion of apical chloride transport in the intestine, although other chloride channels are also active. In fact, Type 2 and Type 3 chloride channels (ClC-2 and ClC-3) are 2 other volume-regulated chloride channels identified in the gastrointestinal tract of both mammalian and non-mammalian cells. Specifically, ClC-2 channels have been found on small and large intestinal epithelial cells and gastrointestinal parietal cells. These chloride channels are involved in a variety of actions including intracellular pH regulation, epithelial chloride transport, and fluid secretion, among other important functions.

Lubiprostone (SPI-0211, RU-0211) was reported to activate apical ClC-2 but not CFTR channels on transfected human cells.[4] As a derivative of a prostaglandin E_1 metabolite, it is classified as a prostone. Unlike prostaglandins, prostones are not thought to stimulate smooth muscle contraction. Figure 38-1 illustrates the postulated mechanism of action of lubiprostone.

In 2009, dispute arose as to lubiprostone's proposed mechanism of action, in particular which chloride channel is stimulated by the drug—the CFTR channel or the ClC-2 channel.[5] Also under debate is whether the drug might directly stimulate smooth muscle through prostaglandin receptors and whether the ClC-2 channel is expressed in the apical

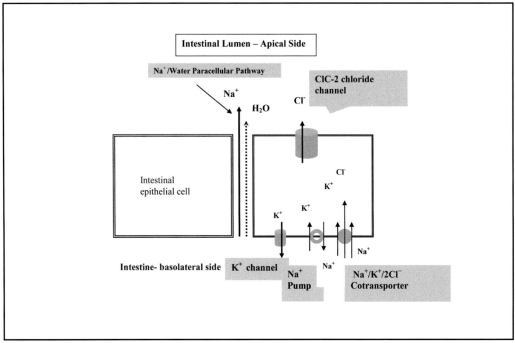

Figure 38-1. Mechanism of action of lubiprostone (Amitiza). The postulated mechanism of action is that the active secretion of chloride from the epithelial ClC-2 channel into the lumen is followed by the passive paracellular secretion of sodium and water resulting in isotonic fluid into the intestinal lumen thereby increasing the liquidity of the intestinal contents. This secretion of fluid is then thought to promote increased intestinal transit, perhaps by stimulation of local stretch receptors resulting in smooth muscle stimulation (Abbreviations: Cl−, chloride, H_2O, Water, K^+, Potassium, Na^+ Sodium).

or basolateral membrane of mucosal epithelium. It appears that the contradictory results may result from disparities in the biophysical properties of the two different chloride channels as well as differences in the concentration of drug used in the different studies. Currently, the evidence favors the drug acting *via* the ClC-2 channel, but further research regarding lubiprostone's influence on CFTR channels and prostaglandin receptors is needed.

In animal studies, lubiprostone has also been shown to stimulate recovery of mucosal barrier function *via* the restoration of tight junction protein complexes. Because mucosal inflammation causing leaky membranes is a proposed mechanism for the development of IBS symptoms in some patients (eg, postinfectious IBS), this finding may have important implications for the drug's role in treating IBS symptoms, although this requires further research.

Although the mechanism of the drug is controversial, its metabolism is more apparent. Unlike many commonly used drugs that rely on the cytochrome P450 system for metabolism (eg, proton pump inhibitors), lubiprostone is metabolized within the GI tract by the microsomal carbonyl reductase system, and therefore less than 0.1% of the drug is actually absorbed. The only measurable active metabolite (M3) is minimally absorbed, and no drug-drug interactions have been reported. Gender has no effect on the drug's metabolism, and elimination of lubiprostone is primarily in the urine and in the feces.

Table 38-1

Bristol Stool Form Scale

Type	Description
1	Separate hard lumps like nuts (difficult to pass)
2	Sausage shaped but lumpy
3	Like sausage but with cracks on its surface
4	Like sausage or snake, smooth and soft
5	Soft blobs with clear cut edges (passed easily)
6	Fluffy pieces with ragged edges, a mushy stool
7	Watery, no solid pieces, entirely liquid

Understanding lubiprostone's place in therapy requires appreciation for the fact that IBS is a chronic disorder with fluctuating symptoms that primarily affects women. IBS is characterized according to the predominant bowel habit—constipation (IBS-C), diarrhea (IBS-D), or mixed type (IBS-M). Treatments are generally focused toward the predominant symptom.[1,2] Treatment of IBS is challenging because, in the natural history of this disorder, bowel habits fluctuate over time. The Rome criteria for IBS (created by a group of gastroenterologists specializing in functional GI disorders) can help to characterize this disorder because the criteria focus on stool characteristics and IBS subtype. For example, patients with IBS-C must have stools that are hard or lumpy more than 25% of the time, and they must be loose or mushy less than 25% of the time. Another tool that can be used to define stool consistency is the Bristol stool scale. Stools are characterized from type 1 (hard lumpy stools) to type 7 (watery stools) (Table 38-1). Last, the clinician must distinguish IBS-C from CIC. Abdominal pain or discomfort is the defining characteristic of IBS-C, but in reality the 2 disorders often overlap in the same individual, which has implications for treatment.

The choice of lubiprostone depends on several factors. First, the effect of traditional lifestyle recommendations, such as increasing fluids, dietary fiber, exercise, and managing stress, needs to be assessed. Clinicians should recognize that there is a paucity of data regarding the effectiveness of these recommendations in IBS patients with moderate to severe disease. Response to conventional medications such as fiber (ispagula husk), antispasmodics (eg, dicyclomine), and osmotic (lactulose and polyethylene glycol 3350) and stimulant laxatives (senna) should be obtained.

Importantly, clinicians need to appreciate the patient's perceived severity of disease. Data exist that IBS patients may be undertreated. A recent online international survey of 1966 patients with IBS using 2 validated instruments to assess severity of disease revealed that 20% to 55% (depending on the instrument used) of these individuals had severe IBS.

Despite the severity of disease in this surveyed population, only about 2% of patients were taking an IBS-targeted drug for their symptoms.

Two double-blind, placebo-controlled studies run in parallel led to the approval of lubiprostone for IBS-C in women 18 years of age or older.[6] The studies randomized 1171 patients (92% women; 92% between the ages of 18 and 65) with IBS-C (using Rome II criteria) to receive lubiprostone 8 mcg or placebo twice daily for 12 weeks. Overall efficacy and safety was evaluated in 1154 adults who completed the 12-week treatment phase of the 2 trials. The overall response rate was calculated based on weekly electronic diary data using the patient's response to a global symptom relief question of how well IBS symptoms were relieved based on a 7-point, balanced Likert symptom relief scale ("significantly worse" to "significantly relieved"). These endpoints represented more rigorous endpoints than had been applied to past clinical trials for IBS, and the response rates were quite low for both the placebo and active drug groups (17.9% versus 10.1%) but were statistically significant. To be an "overall responder," a patient had to be a "monthly responder" for at least 2 of the 3 months of the study. A "monthly responder" was a patient who reported being "significantly relieved" for at least 2 weeks of the month or at least "moderately relieved" in all 4 weeks of that month. In the combined analysis, the overall number needed to treat was approximately 13. A follow-up open-label study assessed the long-term efficacy and safety of lubiprostone. Those patients who initially responded continued to respond during the 48-week trial without any adverse effects not previously reported during the larger 12-week treatment trials. To date, there have been no comparison studies with other options for the treatment of IBS-C.

Research studies have demonstrated that lubiprostone is a safe and effective treatment for IBS-C and can be used as first-line therapy in the treatment of IBS for women 18 years and older (no upper age limit recommended) at the FDA-approved dose of 8 µg twice daily.[3] It is also reasonable in an off-label fashion to start the drug at 8 µg daily with meals and titrate upward to a dose of 24 µg twice daily, if necessary. Realistically, insurance reimbursement often requires that patients fail treatment with PEG or lactulose prior to approving lubiprostone therapy.

Lubiprostone is generally well tolerated, and the chief side effects are nausea, diarrhea, abdominal pain, with rare headache and dyspnea (Table 38-2). Fluid shifts within the gut have been postulated as a possible cause of nausea. Administration of the drug with meals seems to decrease nausea. Data from the constipation studies demonstrated that diarrhea caused no significant change in electrolyte levels over 12 to 48 weeks of treatment. Several patients have described symptoms of dyspnea shortly after taking lubiprostone, although the mechanism by which this occurs is not known. This symptom generally resolved within a few hours, but subsequent doses of the drug caused recurrence of the dyspnea so restarting the drug is not recommended. No electrocardiogram (EKG) changes have been reported in the clinical trials either in constipated patients or in healthy male and female controls. EKG changes were studied after a single 24-µg dose or a supratherapeutic 144-µg dose and did not show any alterations.

In CIC clinical trials, the safety profile of lubiprostone in the elderly ($\geq$ 65 years of age) was consistent with the safety profile in the overall study population. The drug is not yet FDA approved in the pediatric population, but studies are pending. No data are available regarding safety in patients with hepatic or renal impairment.

Table 38-2

Side Effect Profile of Lubiprostone (Amitiza) in IBS-C Clinical Trials

Symptom	Placebo Orally Twice Daily (%) N=435	Lubiprostone Orally 8 ug Twice Daily (%) N=1171
Nausea	4	8
Diarrhea	4	7
Abdominal Pain	2	3
Headache	<1	<1
Dyspnea	Not reported	0.4%

This medication is not recommended in pregnant and lactating women and is classified as pregnancy class C because of its possible association with fetal loss in a single animal study. Again, the mechanism is not known, but is postulated to be related to fluid shifts within the body. Teratogenic effects were not seen in rats and mice, but a small number of guinea pigs receiving supratherapeutic doses of drug developed intrauterine loss. There is no evidence of toxicity in human fetuses to date, but lubiprostone use during pregnancy is advised only if the potential benefit justifies potential risks to the fetus. It is also recommended that women who could become pregnant comply with appropriate contraceptive measures and have a pregnancy test prior to beginning treatment. It is not known whether lubiprostone is secreted into breast milk so, depending on the importance of the drug for the mother, either stopping breastfeeding or stopping the drug is recommended.

Summary

IBS can be a severe and fluctuating disorder for which patients need treatment. Traditional medications may be less effective in delivering global relief, and, until other effective therapies are available for IBS-C data, lubiprostone represents a safe and effective therapy for patients, delivering global relief with minimal side effects.[7]

References

1. Brandt LJ, Chey WD, Foxx-Orenstein AE, et al. An evidence-based systematic review on the management of irritable bowel syndrome. *Am J Gastroenterol.* 2009;104(Suppl 1):S8-S36.
2. Longstreth GF, Thompson WG, Chey WD, Houghton LA, Mearin F, Spiller RC. Functional bowel disorders. *Gastroenterology.* 2006;130(5):1480-1491.

3. AMITIZA (lubiprostone) [Package Insert]. Bethesda, MD: Sucampo Pharmaceuticals, Inc; May 2009.

4. Cuppoletti J, Malinowska DH, Tewari KP, et al. SPI-0211 activates T84 cell chloride transport and recombinant human ClC-2 chloride currents. *Am J Physiol Cell Physiol.* 2004;287(5):C1173-C1183.

5. Bijvelds MJ, Bot AG, Escher JC, De Jonge HR. Activation of intestinal Cl-secretion by lubiprostone requires the cystic fibrosis transmembrane conductance regulator. *Gastroenterology.* 2009;137(3):976-985.

6. Drossman DA, Chey WD, Johanson JF, et al. Clinical trial: lubiprostone in patients with constipation-associated irritable bowel syndrome—results of two randomized, placebo-controlled studies. *Aliment Pharmacol Ther.* 2009;29(3):329-341.

7. Lacy BE, Chey WD. Lubiprostone: chronic constipation and irritable bowel with constipation. *Expert Opin Pharmacother.* 2009;10(1):143-152.

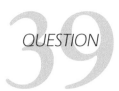
WHAT IS THE ROLE OF ANTIDIARRHEAL AGENTS IN PATIENTS WITH IBS?

Lawrence R. Schiller, MD, FACP, FACG

In the absence of a cure, mitigation of symptoms is the goal of treatment in irritable bowel syndrome (IBS) patients. For patients with IBS with diarrhea, treatment of diarrhea becomes an important management endpoint.[1,2] This is particularly true when diarrhea is accompanied by urgency of defecation or frank fecal incontinence, features that substantially increase the severity of the condition.

Physicians should always remember that diarrhea in IBS can be triggered by environmental issues, such as diet and stress. If possible, these problems should be identified and managed; drug therapy may not be needed if dietary and lifestyle issues are addressed successfully.

When drug therapy is needed, several categories of agents are available: opiates, nonopiate antimotility agents, and stool texture modifiers.

Opiate antidiarrheal drugs have been used to treat diarrhea since antiquity. The agents most commonly used for treating diarrhea, diphenoxylate/atropine and loperamide, are of moderate potency as antidiarrheals, have relatively little central nervous system effect, and are not analgesics. More potent opiates, such as codeine, morphine, and opium, have greater potency as antidiarrheals, but also have important central nervous system effects. These central effects are a double-edged sword. On the one hand, there is an analgesic effect that may mitigate the hallmark symptom of IBS—abdominal pain. On the other hand, there is increased likelihood of habituation and the potential for drug abuse, which are significant issues when managing a chronic painful condition like IBS. Nevertheless, when diarrhea is particularly severe, use of more potent opiates may be necessary.

Opiates work by interacting with μ-opiate receptors in the enteric nervous system to retard gastrointestinal transit.[3] This gives more time for nutrient, fluid, and electrolyte absorption to occur and reduces the amount of luminal contents reaching the rectum. There also are effects on rectal function and sphincter tone that work to improve the reservoir capacity of the rectum. These actions combine to reduce stool weight and stool frequency and to improve urgency and incontinence.

Two trials of loperamide in patients with IBS have been published.[4,5] Both are of relatively short duration and had technical flaws by today's standards for randomized controlled trials. They suggest that loperamide mitigates diarrhea but not abdominal pain or global IBS symptoms. On the basis of these studies, loperamide was felt to be effective for the treatment of diarrhea in IBS by the American College of Gastroenterology Task Force in a recent report.[1]

Opiates should be considered for use in IBS patients with troublesome diarrhea. For some patients, diarrhea is a regular occurrence, and it makes sense to give the antidiarrheal on a scheduled basis. Typical doses are shown in Table 39-1.[2] For other patients, diarrhea is more episodic. If it is predictable—as when diarrhea occurs after a restaurant meal—the antidiarrheal can be taken expectantly, immediately before the trigger. For other patients, diarrhea is more unpredictable; in those patients, opiates can be taken as soon as symptoms develop and may shorten the duration of loose stools.

In general, opiates should be avoided in patients also taking alosetron (see Chapter 40) and should be used cautiously in those with IBS with mixed stool form. In these circumstances, opiates may induce troublesome constipation.

Nonopiate antimotility agents are of 2 types: anticholinergic drugs, such as hyoscyamine, and α_2-adrenergic agonists, such as clonidine.

Anticholinergic drugs are often characterized as antispasmodics, but have important antimotility effects as well. By inhibiting gastric emptying and prolonging intestinal transit, anticholinergic drugs work like opiates to improve net absorption and thereby reduce stool volume. The antidiarrheal effect is less profound than that seen with opiates, though. Side effects of dry mouth and bloating limit patient acceptance, but anticholinergics may be of use in selected patients, particularly those with severe cramping.[6]

Clonidine is an α_2-adrenergic agonist agent ordinarily used for treating hypertension. It has antimotility effects like opiates and also stimulates the rate of intestinal absorption; both of these effects work to mitigate diarrhea.[7] It has been studied as an antidiarrheal drug mostly in patients with diabetic diarrhea. It would likely help diarrhea in patients with IBS, but probably should be used only in IBS patients with concomitant hypertension; unlike diabetics with coexisting autonomic neuropathy (which reduces the antihypertensive effects of clonidine), clonidine might have too much of an antihypertensive effect in normotensive patients.

Stool texture modifiers include resins and polymers that work locally in the gut to affect stool consistency. These include bile acid binding resins and bulking agents, such as fiber and other polymers. They do not necessarily reduce stool weight, but tend to thicken stool.

Bile acid binders, such as cholestyramine, colestipol, and colesevelam, bind up bile acids in the intestine. Because excess bile acid in the colon can cause diarrhea (and this has been postulated as a mechanism for IBS with diarrhea[8]), reducing the concentration below the cathartic threshold may check diarrhea. This situation is most likely to occur after cholecystectomy when bile acids remain in the lumen of the intestine at night and are subject to rapid transfer into the colon when the interdigestive migrating motor complex sweeps through the small intestine. Taking a dose of a bile acid binder at bedtime may mitigate this situation. Bile acid binders may bind other substances in the lumen that may contribute to diarrhea (eg, fatty acids) and modify stool chemistry and bowel function.

Table 39-1
Antidiarrheal Drugs Used in Patients With IBS

Category	Treatment	Typical Adult Dose
Opiate antidiarrheal drugs		
	Diphenoxylate/atropine	1 to 2 tablets QID
	Loperamide	2 to 4 mg QID
	Codeine	15 to 60 mg QID
	Morphine	2 to 20 mg QID
	Deodorized tincture of opium	2 to 10 drops QID
Nonopiate antimotility drugs		
	Hyoscyamine	0.125 to 0.25 mg QID
	Clonidine	0.1 to 0.3 mg TID
Stool texture modifiers: bile acid binders		
	Cholestyramine	4 g hs
	Colestipol	4 g hs
	Colesevelam	2.5 g hs
Stool texture modifiers: bulking agents		
	Psyllium	3 to 6 g up to QID
	Methylcellulose	3 to 6 g up to QID
	Calcium polycarbophil	1.25 g up to QID

Bulking agents are often listed as laxatives, but combine with free water to thicken stools.[9] Psyllium is one of the better-studied agents and can increase stool viscosity when taken in standard doses.[10] Other fiber products and semisynthetic fiber products likely do the same, but have not been studied in depth. One study suggests that calcium polycarbophil modifies stool form when calcium reacts with the polyacrylic acid polymer to form a gel intraluminally. These agents may be of particular help when fecal incontinence is exacerbated by fluid stools; it is easier to retain thicker stools.

References

1. Brandt LJ, Chey WD, Foxx-Orenstein AE, et al. An evidence-based systematic review on the management of irritable bowel syndrome. *Am J Gastroenterol.* 2009;104(Suppl 1):S8-S35.
2. Schiller LR. Management of diarrhea in clinical practice: strategies for primary care physicians. *Rev Gastroenterol Dis.* 2007;7(Suppl 3):S27-S38.
3. Schiller LR, Davis GR, Santa Ana CA, Morawski SG, Fordtran JS. Studies of the mechanism of the antidiarrheal effect of codeine. *J Clin Invest.* 1982;70:999-1008.
4. Hovdenak N. Loperamide treatment of the irritable bowel syndrome. *Scand J Gastroenterol Suppl.* 1987;130:81-84.

5. Lavö B, Stenstam M, Nielsen AL. Loperamide in treatment of irritable bowel syndrome—a double-blind placebo controlled study. *Scand J Gastroenterol Suppl.* 1987;130:77-80.
6. Glende M, Morselli-Labate AM, Battaglia G, Evangelista S. Extended analysis of a double-blind, placebo-controlled, 15-week study with otilonium bromide in irritable bowel syndrome. *Eur J Gastroenterol Hepatol.* 2002;14:1331-1338.
7. Schiller LR, Santa Ana CA, Morawski SG, Fordtran JS. Studies of the antidiarrheal action of clonidine: effects on motility and intestinal absorption. *Gastroenterology.* 1985;89:982-988.
8. Wedlake L, A'Hern R, Russell D, Thomas K, Walters JR, Andreyev HJ. Systematic review: the prevalence of idiopathic bile acid malabsorption as diagnosed by SeHCAT scanning in patients with diarrhoea-predominant irritable bowel syndrome. *Aliment Pharmacol Ther.* 2009;30:707-717.
9. Ford AC, Talley NJ, Spiegel BMR, et al. Effect of fibre, antispasmodics, and peppermint oil in the treatment of irritable bowel syndrome: systematic review and meta-analysis. *BMJ.* 2008;337:a2313.
10. Eherer AJ, Santa Ana CA, Porter J, Fordtran JS. Effect of psyllium, calcium polycarbophil, and wheat bran on secretory diarrhea induced by phenolphthalein. *Gastroenterology.* 1993;104:1007-1012.

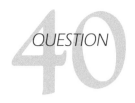
WHAT IS ALOSETRON AND HOW CAN I USE IT?

Brian E. Lacy, MD, PhD

Alosetron (Prometheus Laboratories Inc., San Diego, Calif) is classified as a serotonin (5-HT) receptor antagonist. More specifically, alosetron acts on the 5-HT$_3$ receptor, which is found throughout the enteric neurons in the colon and small intestine, as well as the central nervous system. A number of preclinical studies demonstrated that by blocking the 5-HT$_3$ receptor, alosetron can influence both sensory and motor function of the gastrointestinal (GI) tract. Alosetron slows colonic transit and enhances the reabsorption of fluid from the small intestine, which may lead to an improvement in symptoms of diarrhea. Alosetron has also been shown to improve symptoms of visceral pain, an important factor in the management of IBS patients, because abdominal pain is the most common reason IBS patients seek out consultation. Finally, alosetron improves rectal compliance, which may translate into improvement in symptoms of rectal urgency.[1-3]

Alosetron is rapidly absorbed from the gastrointestinal tract, and serum levels peak approximately 1 to 1.5 hours after ingestion. Concomitant administration with food reduces serum levels by approximately 25%. Alosetron is metabolized by the liver and is excreted renally.

What Is the Efficacy of Alosetron?

A substantial amount of data from multiple, randomized, placebo-controlled clinical trials supports the use of alosetron in women with severe diarrhea-predominant IBS (IBS-D).[3] Two early clinical trials evaluated the efficacy of alosetron in 1273 women with mostly IBS-D or IBS-M (mixed or alternating pattern). All women had IBS symptoms for a minimum of 6 months, and approximately two-thirds of the women were categorized as having IBS-D. In both studies, relief of abdominal pain and discomfort was significantly better in patients treated with alosetron (41% to 43%) than in patients treated with placebo (26% to 29%) after 1, 2, and 3 months of therapy. In both studies, patients treated with alosetron also reported a significant improvement in sensations of rectal urgency, compared to placebo.

Additional data supporting the use of alosetron in women with IBS-D are available from two randomized, double-blind, placebo-controlled trials involving 1293 women.[3] The women in these studies reported frequent bowel urgency, defined as lack of satisfactory control of bowel urgency, for at least 50% of the time for 2 weeks prior to treatment. Alosetron (1 mg orally twice daily) resulted in substantial improvements in the median percentage of days with control of rectal urgency compared to placebo. In addition, daily stool frequency and stool consistency significantly improved in the alosetron group compared with the placebo group ($P<0.001$ for each comparison).

Another study evaluated the effects of three separate doses of alosetron in women with severe IBS-D who had failed conventional therapy and who had symptoms of frequent and severe abdominal pain or discomfort, frequent bowel urgency or fecal incontinence, and/or disability or restriction of daily activities due to their symptoms. A total of 529 women were equally randomized to receive one of three doses of alosetron (0.5 mg qd; 1.0 mg qd; or 1.0 mg bid), while a similar number of patients were randomized to receive placebo. At the end of the 3-month study, women treated with alosetron (all three doses) were more likely to report a significant improvement in IBS symptoms (43% to 51%), using a global improvement scale, compared to those patients treated with placebo (31%; $P\leq0.02$). Analysis of secondary endpoints showed that, at the end of each of the three 4-week treatment intervals, patients treated with alosetron (all 3 doses) were more likely to report an improvement in symptoms of stool consistency ($P\leq0.001$) and stool frequency ($P\leq0.006$), compared with placebo.

Last, the long-term efficacy of alosetron was evaluated in a 48-week multinational, randomized, double-blind study comparing alosetron (1 mg bid) to placebo. Women with IBS-D treated with alosetron reported a greater average rate of adequate relief of IBS pain and discomfort (52% versus 44%; $P=0.01$) and a greater average rate of satisfactory control of bowel urgency (64% versus 52%; $P<0.001$) compared to placebo, respectively. In addition, women with IBS-D noted a significant improvement in symptoms of bowel urgency when treated with alosetron compared to placebo ($P<0.001$). A significant effect was observed as early as after 1 week of treatment, and relief of the symptoms was maintained throughout the treatment period.

Who Is an Appropriate Candidate for Alosetron?

Alosetron is currently the only medication approved by the FDA for the treatment of severe diarrhea-predominant IBS in women (age ≥18 years) who have chronic IBS symptoms (>6 months in duration), who have not responded to conventional therapy, and who do not have any evidence of an anatomic or biochemical abnormality that could explain their symptoms. To further clarify which patients can be treated with alosetron, the Food and Drug Administration has stated that, to be categorized as a "severe" IBS with diarrhea patient, women must meet *just* one of three of the following criteria: frequent and severe abdominal pain/discomfort; **or** frequent bowel urgency or fecal incontinence; **or** disability or restriction of daily activities due to IBS. In clinical practice, this means that if a woman has symptoms of IBS-D for more than 6 months and has not responded adequately to conventional therapy (eg, dietary changes, Imodium), then the patient is a candidate for alosetron. In my experience, I believe that alosetron is unfortunately reserved for only the most severe IBS patient who has failed every imaginable medical therapy available. This means that appropriate treatment is often delayed for women who remain symptomatic with IBS-D symptoms. This is unfortunate, because delaying appropriate treatment contributes to continued impairments in quality of life. Thus, I recommend that, given the strong evidence available to date supporting its use, alosetron be used earlier for women with severe IBS-D who have not responded to conventional therapy.

Is There Anything I Should Be Concerned About When I Prescribe Alosetron?

Alosetron has a unique marketing history. It was first approved by the US Food and Drug Administration for the treatment of women with IBS-D in February 2000 and reached US markets 2 months later. Due to concerns over a possible association with serious complications of constipation and ischemic colitis, alosetron was voluntarily withdrawn from the US market in November 2000. In June 2002, the drug was returned to the market by the FDA for women with severe IBS-D who had failed standard therapy. Since then, alosetron has been available for women with IBS-D only through physicians who have enrolled in a risk management plan (RMP). Of note, since the RMP was introduced, the number of serious adverse events has dropped significantly (see below).

In clinical trials, the most common adverse event associated with alosetron use has been constipation, observed in 29% of all IBS patients treated with alosetron versus 6% who received placebo ($P<0.0001$). Adverse GI events occurring in at least 1% of IBS patients receiving alosetron or placebo are shown in Table 40-1. Note that only constipation occurred at a significantly greater rate than placebo. Constipation appears to be a dose-related side effect. For the majority of patients who experienced constipation, it was rated as mild and was self-limited in nature, especially when the dose medication was reduced or stopped. Non-GI adverse events reported in 3% or more of patients receiving alosetron or placebo and occurring more frequently with alosetron than placebo included upper respiratory tract infection, muscle spasms, headaches, and fatigue.

The 2 most worrisome serious adverse events associated with alosetron are complications of constipation and ischemic colitis. The rate of serious complications of constipation in clinical trials was found to range from 0.36 to 0.95 per 1000 patient-years, depending upon the level of evidence available to support a possible association. Serious adverse events that have occurred with severe constipation include bowel obstruction, ileus, impaction, toxic megacolon, perforation, and intestinal ulceration. Although frequently discussed, the rate of ischemic colitis is actually quite low and was recently calculated at 0.95 to 1.25 cases per 1000 patient-years. This appears to be an idiosyncratic reaction and is not dose related.[2] Interestingly, since the initial reports of adverse events associated with alosetron were published, research has shown that all patients with IBS are at a two- to fourfold increased risk for ischemic colitis compared to the general population.[4] It is thus quite possible that some of the initial adverse events attributed to alosetron were in fact due to the underlying disorder and not the medication. Nonetheless, alosetron currently carries a black box warning for infrequent but serious GI adverse reactions, including ischemic colitis and serious complications of constipation.

Table 40-1

Summary of Adverse Events From Alosetron Clinical Trials (22 Clinical Trials Involving 1 mg bid Alosetron versus Placebo)

Adverse Event	Alosetron, % Patients (n=8328)	Placebo, % Patients (n=2363)
Constipation	29	6
Abdominal discomfort and pain	7	4
Nausea	6	5
Gastrointestinal discomfort and pain	5	3
Abdominal distention	2	1
Regurgitation and reflux	2	2
Hemorrhoids	2	1

Note that constipation was the only adverse effect found to be satistically significant when comparing rates of adverse events between patients treated with alosetron versus placebo.

How Do I Use Alosetron?

The first step for physicians interested in prescribing alosetron for their female patients with severe IBS-D is to enroll in the Prescribing Program. This form takes just a few minutes to complete. Physicians must then provide the appropriate patient with a medication guide that is included in the Prescribing Program guidebook. Both patient and physician must then sign a Patient-Physician Agreement form before treatment is begun. A special sticker must also be applied to the prescription, which alerts the pharmacist to the Prescribing Program. Alosetron tablets are available in 2 different doses, 0.5-mg and 1-mg tablets. The FDA recommends that alosetron be started at 0.5 mg orally twice daily. In my practice, however, I tend to start all appropriate patients on a lower daily dose. In general, I prescribe 0.5 mg each day as the starting dose, taken 1 to 1.5 hours before the time of day when their worst IBS-D symptoms develop. I remind patients to watch for warning signs of severe constipation and ischemic colitis (abdominal pain, hematochezia, and diarrhea), and I ask them to call 7 to 10 days after treatment is initiated. If their IBS-D symptoms have improved significantly, I have them continue the same dose and return for a follow-up visit in 3 to 4 weeks. If they have not had any improvement, then I will increase the dose to 0.5 mg twice daily and again ask them to call back for follow-up 7 to 10 days later. Over the next several weeks, if symptoms remain persistent (and warning signs are absent), then I will have them slowly increase the dose to 1 mg orally twice daily. If they do not notice any improvement in IBS-D symptoms after 4 to 6 continuous weeks of 1 mg alosetron taken twice daily, then I will stop the medication. If patients notice some improvement in symptoms and have not had any side effects, then I will continue alosetron but will consider adding an additional medication, such as a tricyclic antidepressant (if abdominal pain remains an issue), a probiotic (if bloating remains an issue), or Imodium or diphenoxylate-atropine (if diarrhea persists). In patients who develop constipation, I generally ask them to stop their alosetron until the symptoms resolve and then restart alosetron at a lower dose. I have found this step-wise approach to be quite effective and safe.

Summary

A recent systematic review and meta-analysis of eight randomized controlled trials involving 4987 patients determined that alosetron provided a significant reduction in the global symptoms of diarrhea, abdominal pain, and bloating in patients with IBS and diarrhea.[5] Unfortunately, many women with IBS-D are inappropriately labeled as having only mild symptoms and, thus, are not offered therapy with a medication that has been shown to improve global IBS-D symptoms and that can significantly improve quality of life.[6] This is unfortunate, because undertreatment of IBS-D symptoms may lead to unnecessary office visits and scheduling of unnecessary, expensive tests, some of which are associated with significant risks.

References

1. Chang L, Tong K, Ameen V. Ischemic colitis and complications of constipation associated with the use of alosetron under a risk management plan: clinical characteristics, outcomes, and incidences. *Am J Gastroenterol.* 2010;105(4):866-875.
2. Chey WD, Chey WY, Heath AT, et al. Long-term safety and efficacy of alosetron in women with severe diarrhea-predominant irritable bowel syndrome. *Am J Gastroenterol.* 2004;99:2195-2203.
3. Ford AC, Brandt LJ, Young C, et al. Efficacy of 5-HT3 antagonists and 5-HT4 agonists in irritable bowel syndrome: systematic review and meta-analysis. *Am J Gastroenterol.* 2009;104:1831-1843.
4. Higgins PD, Davis KJ, Laine L. Systematic review: the epidemiology of ischaemic colitis. *Aliment Pharmacol Ther.* 2004;19:729-738.
5. Rahimi R, Nikfar S, Abdollahi M. Efficacy and tolerability of alosetron for the treatment of irritable bowel syndrome in women and men: a meta-analysis of eight randomized, placebo-controlled 12-week trials. *Clin Ther.* 2008;30:884-901.
6. Lembo A, Ameen VZ, Drossman DA. Irritable bowel syndrome: toward an understanding of severity. *Clin Gastroenterol Hepatol.* 2005;3:717-725.

WHAT ARE PROBIOTICS AND DO THEY WORK IN IBS?

Yehuda Ringel, MD

Probiotics are live microorganisms that, when administered in adequate amount, confer a health benefit to the host.[1] Commonly used probiotic bacteria include strains of lactic acid bacilli (*Lactobacillus, Bifidobacterium, Lactococcus*), other nonpathogenic strains of bacteria (*E. coli Nissle* 1917, *Clostridium butyricum, Streptococcus thermophilus, Streptococcus salivarius, Bacillus coagulans,* and *Enterococcus faecium*), and nonpathogenic strains of yeast (*Saccharomyces boulardii* and *Saccharomyces cerevisiae*).

Probiotics may be found in certain food products, such as yogurts and fermented milk, bars, cereals, and baby formulas, or in over-the-counter preparations in the form of capsules, pills, and powders. In general, the amount of the probiotic bacteria is usually lower in probiotic foods than in prescribed and over-the-counter probiotic products. However, many of the marketed probiotic foods include additional food ingredients that can selectively promote the growth or function of probiotic bacteria in the intestine (ie, prebiotics). Thus, the combination of *probiotics* and *prebiotics* (often referred to as *synbiotics*) in certain food products may further increase, at least theoretically, the beneficial effects of these products.

Probiotics can be categorized as foods, dietary supplements, or drugs depending on how they are used and labeled. From the US Food and Drug Administration (FDA) perspective, if a probiotic is used to cure, treat, prevent, or mitigate a disease condition, it should be considered a drug. However, currently in the United States, probiotic products are available only as food and dietary supplements and as such do not require FDA approval for marketing.

The concept of using probiotic microbes to improve the characteristics of the intestinal microbiota and promote health is not a new idea. Microbiologic organisms in various cultures have been used to process food (eg, by fermentation) for many years as a way to store perishable food and improve taste. More than 100 years ago, the Nobel Prize-winning microbiologist Elie Metchnikoff (1845-1919) hypothesized that the consumption of yogurts fermented with *Lactobacillus* was responsible for the increased longevity of Bulgarian peasants.

The mechanisms by which probiotics may promote health are not completely understood but may include suppression of growth or epithelial binding of pathogenic bacteria; improvement of intestinal barrier function; modulation of the mucosal immune system; assistance with digestion and absorption of nutrients, vitamins, and minerals; synthesis of nutritional elements from sources the human body is not able to use; and/or production of byproducts that benefit the host.

The rationale for using probiotics in irritable bowel syndrome (IBS) is based on the idea that the normal composition of the intestinal bacteria (also called *intestinal microbiota*) is important in maintaining normal functioning of the intestinal tract and that disruption of the intestinal microbiota may lead to alterations in intestinal function and functional GI symptoms. Several epidemiologic and microbiology findings support this hypothesis. Examples include the development of long-lasting GI symptoms following acute bacterial gastroenteritis (ie, *postinfectious IBS* or the presence of small intestinal bacterial overgrowth). Recent microbiology studies indicate that the composition of the intestinal microbiota in patients with IBS is different than in healthy people. However, because of the complexity of the intestinal microbiota and the fact that most of the bacteria in the human intestine are still unknown, the specific alterations are not yet well characterized. In addition, it is not yet clear whether these recently described differences are the cause for IBS symptoms or a secondary result of the abnormal intestinal function in these patients.[2]

Clinical Use of Probiotics in IBS

Early studies relating to the clinical use of probiotics as a treatment for IBS have shown mixed results and have exhibited considerable methodological limitations.[3-5] However, more recent studies that have employed sound methodologies provided more solid data and suggested possible benefits for the use of certain probiotics in the treatment of IBS.

Although a number of probiotic bacteria have been tested in patients with IBS and have been shown to be beneficial in alleviating global or individual symptoms of IBS (eg, pain/discomfort, bloating, flatulence, and constipation), very few products have been tested in their final formulation in these patients. Only a few studies have investigated the physiologic effects of probiotics in IBS. These studies have shown that a probiotic yogurt containing *Bifidobacterium animalis* DN-173-010 and a synbiotic yogurt containing the probiotic bacterium *Bifidobacterium animalis* ssp. *lactis* Bb12 and the prebiotic inulin have an accelerating effect on colonic transit, whereas a probiotic mixture of 8 species of bacteria (VSL#3) has an opposite effect of delaying colonic transit compared with placebo. These studies demonstrate that probiotics can affect specific aspects of intestinal physiology (eg, intestinal transit time) relevant to functional GI disorders and that these effects may be strain-specific.

The clinical effects of probiotics in IBS have been evaluated in only a relatively small number of clinical trials. A review of the published literature reveals an overall paucity of high-quality studies and difficulties in comparing and summarizing the data (eg, by meta-analysis) due to differences in the probiotic strains, dose, and study design. Nevertheless, recent systematic reviews concluded that probiotics appear to be efficacious in IBS, although the magnitude of benefit and the most effective species and strain are uncertain.[3-5]

It is important to recognize that not all probiotics are the same and not all marketed probiotic products actually contain probiotic strains at efficacious concentrations. In addition, most of the available products were not clinically tested in patients with IBS. Thus, when considering which probiotic product to recommend to a patient, an important criterion should be whether the probiotic product was tested, in its final formulation, for that particular condition.

Summary

Recent studies support the idea that the intestinal microbiota play a role in the pathogenesis of IBS and that manipulation of the intestinal microbiota by probiotics may be beneficial in improving relevant GI functions and reducing GI symptoms in some patients with IBS. However, the overall beneficial effects of probiotics seem to be modest, the mechanisms by which probiotics induce their beneficial effects is unclear, and the association between probiotics-induced microbiology and physiologic effects and the clinical improvement in IBS symptoms needs to be proven.

References

1. Guarner F, Schaafsma GJ. Short communication: probiotics. *Int J Food Microbiol.* 1998;39:237-238.
2. Ringel Y, Carroll IM. Alterations in the intestinal microbiota and functional bowel symptoms. *Gastrointest Endosc Clin N Am.* 2009;19(1):141-150.
3. Brenner DM, Moeller MJ, Chey WD, Schoenfeld PS. The utility of probiotics in the treatment of irritable bowel syndrome: a systematic review. *Am J Gastroenterol.* 2009;104(4):1033-1049.
4. Hoveyda N, Heneghan C, Mahtani KR, Perera R, Roberts N, Glasziou P. A systematic review and meta-analysis: probiotics in the treatment of irritable bowel syndrome. *BMC Gastroenterol.* 2009;9:15.
5. Moayyedi P, Ford AC, Talley NJ, et al. The efficacy of probiotics in the treatment of irritable bowel syndrome: a systematic review. *Gut.* 2010;59(3):325-332.

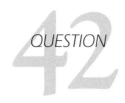

WHICH PROBIOTICS ARE BEST FOR PATIENTS WITH IBS?

Eamonn M. M. Quigley, MD, FRCP, FACP, FACG, FRCPI

The first response of a busy clinician to the question, "Which probiotics are best for patients with IBS?" is a much more direct and basic one: "Why even consider a probiotic?"

This question can be answered on a number of levels. At the most basic level, the current interest in probiotics in the medical community (in contrast to the general public who have been happily consuming "probiotic" products for decades) reflects the belated recognition of the importance of the gut flora (or, more correctly, microbiota) to man. Indeed, it is now abundantly evident that the enteric microbiota influences a variety of intestinal functions and plays a key role in nutrition, in maintaining the integrity of the epithelial barrier, and in the development of mucosal immunity. Simultaneously, the true extent of the consequences of disturbances in the microbiota or in its interaction with the host to health has been recognized. Some of these are relatively obvious and are seen on an all-too-frequent basis in your practice: antibiotic-associated diarrhea and its deadliest manifestation, *Clostridium difficile* colitis, as a consequence of antibiotic use, or small intestinal bacterial overgrowth in the context of altered anatomy, impaired motility, or diminished acid secretion. More subtle qualitative or quantitative changes in the microbiota and/or in its interaction with the host seem likely to be relevant to a large number of gastrointestinal disorders, ranging from the many manifestations of *Helicobacter pylori* infection to inflammatory bowel disease and even obesity. With the description of the ability of enteric infections to trigger the onset of IBS in susceptible individuals, the documentation of immune activation in the intestinal mucosa and in the systemic immune compartment, as well as a suggestion that all may not be well in the lumen in terms of the microbiota in IBS, this disorder has now joined the list of conditions associated with alterations in the gut microbiota. A role for enteric bacteria in IBS has been bolstered, of course, by reports of clinical responses to antibiotic therapy. So this provides a very general rationale for considering a probiotic in IBS, but what is the evidence?

Until the year 2000, a small number of studies evaluated the response of IBS to probiotic preparations, and, while results between studies were difficult to compare because of differences in study design, probiotic dose, and strain, there was some, but by no means consistent, evidence of symptom improvement.[1] Further studies, since then, have assessed the response to a number of well-characterized organisms and have produced discernible trends.[1] Indeed, a number of recent meta-analyses have concluded that probiotics, in general, do benefit patients with IBS.[2,3] What are more difficult to define are the relative benefits of different species or strains. In one of these meta-analyses, for example, it was concluded that *Bifidobacteria*, as a species, were effective in IBS while *Lactobacilli* were not.[2] A major problem facing any analyst of the literature in this field continues to be the poor quality of many studies: small study populations, variable end-points, and the use of various organisms bedevil their interpretation. Indeed, Brenner and colleagues went so far as to state that only one organism, *Bifidobacterium infantis* 35624, had support for efficacy in IBS based on clinical studies of adequate quality.[3] Since that publication, another strain, *Bifidobacterium lactis* DN-173-010A, has shown particular promise among IBS subjects with constipation-predominant IBS and prominent bloating. Indeed, the clinical effects of this strain on constipation and bloating have been supported by evidence that this bacterium accelerates colon transit and reduces abdominal distension. Well, it sounds as if it is worth trying a probiotic in IBS, so what do I say to my patient when she asks me about a product that she has picked up in a health food store?

Probiotics are defined as live organisms that, when ingested in adequate amounts, exert a health benefit to the host. Over the years, many products have appeared on health food store and supermarket shelves throughout the world that include the term probiotic in their label. Very few fulfill the definition provided:

1. They may not contain live organisms or have not been adequately tested to ensure that the organisms will survive in the conditions (eg, room temperature) or for the length of time (days, weeks, or months) that is claimed.

2. They may not confer any health benefit because, either they have never been tested in man or the studies that have been performed have been inadequate or even negative.

Other issues of quality control continue to complicate the probiotic area. Does the product actually contain the organism and the dose of that organism that the label claims that it contains? Unfortunately, when researchers have analyzed some store products, they have found, not only that organisms claimed to be alive were actually dead, but that the product contained organisms (including pathogens) that it was not supposed to contain. The good news is that some companies producing probiotics have gone to considerable efforts to ensure that their products do contain the very organisms and in the precise dose that are claimed. These products can guarantee the survival of live organisms over the time and in the conditions specified on the label. Whether or not these same products can provide the health benefits that they claim can only be deduced from a critical assessment of the medical literature. This is currently not a very satisfactory situation for the patient and his or her doctor. Indeed, until adequate regulation is introduced into this field, the best advice that you can give to your patient is to tell him or her to stick with reputable manufacturers. Next, he or she asks the killer question: Does it matter which probiotic I use?

Just as no 2 drugs are identical, no 2 probiotics are the same! Even within the same species, different strains may have vastly different and even contrasting effects, and this has been amply demonstrated in numerous tests of antibacterial, antiviral, metabolic, and immunological effects of these bugs. Differences are now emerging from clinical studies. Even in IBS, as described above, while it has been shown that probiotics, in general, seem to have an effect; in many instances, these benefits are limited to individual symptoms, such as bloating, diarrhea, or constipation, and very few have been shown to demonstrate global benefits in IBS. Some have worked only among IBS sub-groups: diarrhea-predominant, constipation-predominant, prominent bloaters; a few seem to benefit all IBS groups to some extent. Furthermore, none of the strains available in the US have been subjected to long-term study, a critical deficit in a condition as chronic and recurrent as IBS.

I share all this information with the patient, suggest that a high-quality *Bifidobacterium*, such as *Bifidobacterium infantis* 35624, seems to have the edge right now, but he or she has one last and even more difficult question: Are probiotics safe?

Many different species and strains and preparations of probiotics have been used for decades and by millions of healthy and diseased individuals, yet definitive data on safety are scanty. Overall, however, the safety record is very good, and reports of sepsis are rare.[4] Even then, the evidence incriminating the probiotic organism administered as the source of a given instance of sepsis is weak. For the moment, it seems prudent to use probiotics with caution in certain patient groups—particularly neonates born prematurely, with immune deficiency, or with the short bowel syndrome. A scare was generated recently by a report of increased mortality among patients with severe acute pancreatitis who had been administered a probiotic cocktail through a naso-enteric tube. These deaths were associated not with sepsis, but with intestinal ischemia whose etiology remains unclear. None of these are relevant to IBS, fortunately, so you can be reassuring about safety.

The bottom line: probiotics and some strains in particular may well help your IBS patient. They are safe and certainly worth a try.

References

1. Quigley EMM, Flourie B. Probiotics in irritable bowel syndrome: a rationale for their use and an assessment of the evidence to date. *Neurogastroenterol Motil.* 2007;19:166-172.
2. Moayyedi P, Ford AC, Talley NJ, et al. The efficacy of probiotics in the therapy of irritable bowel syndrome: a systematic review. *Gut.* 2010;59:325-332.
3. Brenner DM, Moeller MJ, Chey WD, Schoenfeld PS. The utility of probiotics in the treatment of irritable bowel syndrome: A systematic review. *Am J Gastroenterol.* 2009;104:1033-1049.
4. Boyle RJ, Robins-Browne RM, Tang MLK. Probiotic use in clinical practice: what are the risks? *Am J Clin Nutr.* 2006;83:1256-1264.

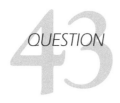

LINACLOTIDE—WHAT IS IT AND WHY MIGHT IT HELP MY PATIENTS WITH IBS?

Burr Loew, MD and Brian E. Lacy, MD, PhD

Linaclotide (Ironwood Pharmaceuticals, Cambridge, Mass) is a 14-amino acid peptide that stimulates intestinal guanylate cyclase-type-C (GC-C) receptors. Linaclotide is acid stable and protease resistant. In addition, bioavailability is low, meaning that most of the medication remains within the gastrointestinal (GI) tract; it is undetectable in the systemic circulation at therapeutic doses. Linaclotide mimics the action of endogenous guanylin (15 amino acids) and uroguanylin (16 amino acids), both of which activate the GC-C receptor. Guanylate cyclase-C is expressed at high levels in the small intestine and colon, but low levels in the stomach. Activation of GC-C stimulates the production of cyclic guanosine monophosphate (cGMP) from guanosine triphosphate (GTP), which then increases the flow of electrolytes (HCO_3^- and Cl^-) and water into the lumen of the GI tract, leading to a reflexive increase in GI transit. In addition, stimulation of the GC-C receptor on intestinal epithelial cells and release of cGMP into the serosa leads to a reduction in visceral hyperalgesia.

What Is the Evidence from Preclinical Trials That Linaclotide Might Help IBS Patients?

Early animal studies in mice and rats showed that linaclotide increased intestinal fluid secretion and stimulated intestinal transit more than placebo or tegaserod (a 5-HT4 agonist that was used to treat chronic constipation [CC] and IBS with constipation [IBS-C]; tegaserod is not currently available in the United States). The beneficial effects of linaclotide on intestinal transit were lost in GC-C receptor knockout mice, demonstrating the specificity of linaclotide for this receptor. Two different animal models from two different laboratories demonstrated that linaclotide suppressed visceral hyperalgesia and colorectal allodynia. Finally, tissue culture studies demonstrated that linaclotide binds to GC-C receptors on human colon cells and stimulates cGMP production. These results led to phase 1 dose ranging and pharmacodynamic studies in healthy human volunteers and, subsequently, phase II studies as described below, as well as ongoing phase III trials.

What Clinical Data Are Available Showing That Linaclotide Might Help Patients with Constipation?

Johnston and colleagues were the first to investigate the safety, tolerability, and efficacy of linaclotide in patients with CC who met modified Rome II criteria.[1] In this multicenter, placebo-controlled pilot study, 42 patients were randomized to one of three doses of linaclotide (100, 300, or 1000 µg) or placebo once daily for 2 weeks. On a daily basis for the 7 days preceding therapy and then during treatment, patients recorded daily bowel habits, including stool frequency, consistency according to the Bristol Stool Form Scale (BSFS), straining and completeness of evacuation, and subjective patient-reported outcomes (ie, abdominal discomfort, overall relief, and severity of constipation). Given the small sample size, the study endpoints were not intended to achieve statistical significance; however, there was a trend toward a dose-dependent increase in frequency of weekly spontaneous bowel movements (SBMs) and complete spontaneous bowel movements (CSBMs). Stool consistency, straining, and patient-reported outcomes also improved in all dosing groups. Twenty-two adverse events (AEs) were reported in 13 of 42 patients (30%) without significant difference among all the groups. All AEs were mild-moderate in severity and mostly GI in nature. Diarrhea was the most common side effect, occurring in 13% of all study drug patients, but without a noticeable dose-dependent effect. No patient treated with placebo reported diarrhea as an AE. These promising results led to a larger phase II study as described below.

A large multicenter, placebo-controlled study evaluated 310 patients with CC as defined by modified Rome II criteria.[2] Patients were randomized to 1 of 4 linaclotide dosages (75, 150, 300, or 600 µg) or placebo once daily for 4 weeks. The primary endpoint was the change in mean weekly SBM frequency from the 14-day pretreatment period to the 4-week treatment period. Lembo and colleagues noted that the frequency of weekly SBMs increased significantly in a linear response to increasing dosages of linaclotide (2.6, 3.3, 3.6, and 4.3 for linaclotide doses of 75, 150, 300, and 600 µg, respectively) compared to 1.5 for placebo ($P<0.05$ for each linaclotide dosage group compared to placebo). The median time to first SBM, mean number of CSBMs, stool consistency, and severity of straining also demonstrated a significantly improved dose-dependent relationship compared to placebo. Subjective patient measures including abdominal discomfort, bloating, global measures of constipation, and health-related quality of life were significantly better for all linaclotide dosing regimens compared to placebo. During a 14-day post-treatment surveillance period, bowel habits were noted to trend toward baseline, suggesting that linaclotide does not cause a rebound worsening of constipation symptoms. Adverse events were reported in 33.8% of patients receiving the study drug and in 31.9% of placebo (ns). The most commonly reported AEs were GI-related, of which diarrhea was the most frequent (5.1%, 8.9%, 4.8%, and 14.3% in the 75, 150, 300, and 600 µg groups, respectively) versus 2.9% of placebo patients. Only 2 cases of diarrhea were graded as severe. Both were in the 600-µg group, and both resulted in cessation of treatment. Although these studies included only about 10% men and less than 20% non-Whites, linaclotide appears to as be equally effective in these subgroups as the intention-to-treat population.

What Data Are Available Showing That Linaclotide Might Help My Patient With IBS With Constipation?

The first study to evaluate the safety and efficacy of linaclotide in patients with IBS-C involved 36 women who met Rome II criteria for IBS-C.[3] During the baseline period, symptoms were measured, the BSFS completed, and colonic transit measured. Patients were then randomized equally to either placebo or one of two doses of linaclotide (100 or 1000 µg daily) for a 5-day treatment period. Symptoms were measured during the treatment period, and colonic transit was again measured. Andresen and colleagues reported that the 1000-µg daily dose of linaclotide, but not the 100-µg daily dose, improved ascending colon filling more than placebo ($P=0.015$) and also accelerated overall colonic transit at 48 hours ($P=0.01$). Linaclotide did not affect gastric emptying at either dose. Compared to placebo, both the 100-µg daily dose and the 1000-µg daily dose of linaclotide improved stool frequency, stool consistency, and the time to first bowel movement. No serious AEs were noted, and there was no difference in AEs between linaclotide and placebo. Although the sample size of this pilot study was small, these encouraging results led to the initiation of a much larger phase II study, described below.

The trial by Johnston and colleagues was designed as a multicenter, double-blind, placebo-controlled, dose-ranging study involving 420 patients with IBS-C (modified Rome II criteria; <3 CSBMs/week).[4] Patients were randomized to one of four different daily doses of linaclotide (75, 150, 300, or 600 µg) or placebo for 12 weeks after a 2-week baseline period where symptoms were monitored. The primary endpoint was the change in CSBM frequency, while other bowel symptoms (eg, straining and consistency) as well as abdominal symptoms (eg, abdominal pain and bloating) were secondary endpoints. Three-hundred and thirty-seven patients (80%) completed the entire study; 13 patients on the study medication, but none on placebo, discontinued the study due to significant diarrhea. Routine monitoring did not reveal any evidence of electrolyte abnormalities or dehydration. Using a strict intention-to-treat analysis (where patients who dropped out were considered treatment failures), linaclotide at all study doses was shown to significantly improve stool frequency ($P<0.023$ or better for all doses), in addition to symptoms of straining, bloating, and abdominal pain (all with $P<0.05$ except for bloating using the 150-µg dose, which was not statistically better than placebo). In addition, patients treated with linaclotide (all doses) were more likely than those treated with placebo to report adequate relief of global IBS symptoms for at least 6 weeks of the 12-week treatment period. Cessation of the study medication at the end of the trial did not appear to lead to a worsening of IBS symptoms (ie, no rebound effect was noted). At the time of publication of this book, these results are still in abstract form. However, these promising results led to the initiation of two large phase III clinical trials, which are currently ongoing.

These studies are evaluating the efficacy and safety of linaclotide in patients with IBS-C. Both studies, which are available only in abstract form at the time of this book's publication, were designed as multicenter, randomized, double-blind, placebo-controlled trials. The first study involved 803 patients who met Rome II criteria for IBS-C. Symptoms were measured for 2 weeks before drug randomization, and during this time, 88% of all patients had abdominal pain every day. Patients were then randomized to either linaclotide (266 µg once daily) or placebo for 12 weeks. All patients were also followed during a 4-week withdrawal period. Using recommendations from the FDA draft guidance published in March 2010, one composite responder endpoint evaluated both abdominal pain and CSBM. To meet criteria as a responder, patients had to have a 30% reduction in abdominal pain and an increase of at least one CSBM per week, for at least 6 of 12 treatment weeks. Patients randomized to linaclotide were much more likely to meet this endpoint (33.6%) compared to those randomized to placebo (21%; $P<0.0001$). Using even more strict criteria of having a 30% reduction in abdominal pain, at least three CSBMs, and an increase of at least one CSBM for at least 9 of 12 weeks, patients randomized to linaclotide (12.1%) were more likely to reach this high bar compared to those randomized to placebo (5.1%; $P<0.0004$). Although these results seem less impressive than other IBS studies, it is critical to keep in mind that the criteria used to judge a patient as a responder were the strictest criteria ever used in an IBS research study. Finally, results of the second randomized, placebo-controlled study, which involved 805 patients, were slightly better than the first study, which supports the view that linaclotide will prove beneficial at treating IBS patients with constipation.

Summary

Chronic constipation and IBS with constipation are highly prevalent conditions that significantly impair patients' quality of life. Traditional treatments such as lifestyle modifications, fiber supplementation, smooth muscle relaxants, and laxatives are often prescribed, although their effectiveness is often limited. In our experience, patients with significant or refractory symptoms are often frustrated by their lack of improvement with these measures and are desperate for alternative treatment modalities. Many patients would gladly consider other therapeutic options even if the benefits were expected to be low and the risks of AEs thought to be high. Despite their prevalence, only a few medications for these disorders have been FDA-approved. Tegaserod, a 5-HT4 partial agonist, was removed from the market in 2007 because of concerns of increased risks for cardiovascular events. Lubiprostone, a locally acting chloride channel activator, was approved for the treatment of CC in adults and IBS-C in women and has been shown to improve symptoms in many patients. However, nausea is a bothersome side effect in some patients, which may lead to drug discontinuation. As described above, linaclotide, a novel therapeutic agent with specificity for the GC-C receptor located in the small intestine and colon, appears to be a highly effective treatment for patients with CC and IBS-C. The robust efficacy seen in these preliminary clinical trials, overall patient satisfaction, lack of systemic side effects, and limited AEs are exciting findings and are unique among currently available agents. The preliminary results of phase III trials appear quite promising, and we are hopeful that this medication will provide a needed treatment option for patients with refractory symptoms to standard treatments.

References

1. Johnston JM, Kurtz CB, Drossman DA, et al. Pilot study of the effect of linaclotide in patients with chronic constipation. *Am J Gastroenterol*. 2009;104:125-132.
2. Lembo AJ, Kurtz CB, MacDougall JE, et al. Efficacy of linaclotide for patients with chronic constipation. *Gastroenterology*. 2010;138:886-895.
3. Andresen V, Camilleri M, Busciglio IA, et al. Effect of 5 days linaclotide on transit and bowel function in females with constipation-predominant irritable bowel syndrome. *Gastroenterology*. 2007;133:761-768.
4. Johnston JM, Kurtz CB, MacDougall JE, et al. Linaclotide improves abdominal pain and bowel habits in a Phase IIb study of patients with irritable bowel syndrome with constipation. *Gastroenterology*. 2010;139:1877-1886.

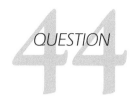
WILL ACUPUNCTURE HELP MY PATIENTS WITH IBS?

Elizabeth A. Friedlander, PhD, ANP-C, FNP and Anthony Lembo, MD

Acupuncture, an ancient traditional Chinese medical practice, is becoming more widely accepted and used in Western society.[1] Traditional Chinese medicine is based on a theory of energy or life force ("qi") that runs through the body in 14 channels called meridians and regulates all physical and mental processes in the body. In theory, the meridians run deep within the body but surface at more than 360 places (acupuncture points). Qi is essential to health, and disruptions of this flow, which are believed to contribute to symptoms and diseases, can be corrected at identifiable anatomical locations ("acupoints") with acupuncture. Acupuncture is most commonly used to reduce pain and nausea; its role in irritable bowel syndrome (IBS) has not been well studied and remains unclear.

Acupuncture has the potential to improve IBS symptoms through several different mechanisms, including alteration in gut visceral sensation and motility and stimulation of the somatic nervous system and vagus nerve. The latter occurs through the release of endogenous endorphins, serotonin, norepinephrine, and prostaglandins. A Cochrane database review of published studies prior to 2006 found 6 randomized clinical trials using acupuncture in IBS. The studies were generally of poor quality, included relatively small numbers of patients, and differed significantly in acupuncture method used (standardized vs individualized). Limitations notwithstanding, the review found inconclusive evidence as to whether acupuncture is superior to sham (placebo) acupuncture in IBS. Likewise, a systematic review published in 2007 also concluded that there was insufficient evidence that acupuncture was superior to sham acupuncture (Table 44-1). The authors of this review suggested that sham acupuncture may not be an adequate placebo.

Several well-conducted studies evaluating the effects of acupuncture in IBS have recently been published. Schneider and colleagues published a well-conducted study in which 43 IBS patients were randomized to 10 acupuncture treatment sessions using 8 acupoints over 5 weeks or sham acupuncture. There was no significant difference between the response rates in patients receiving acupuncture and sham acupuncture on a specific quality-of-life measurement for functional bowel digestive disorders (FBDDQL), although patients in both groups improved significantly compared to baseline. In another

Table 44-1

Clinical Trials of Acupuncture in IBS

Reference	Study Design	Treatment	n	Duration of Treatment	Primary Outcome	Results
Ref. 4	RCT with re-randomization at 3 weeks. Sectional evaluation.	Six fixed and 11 optional acupoints in augmented or limited patient interaction vs wait list control	230	Six treatments 3 weeks after 3-week "run in" with sham	IBS-GIS; IBS-SSS; IBS-AR; IBS-QOL	No difference between sham and AC. Both superior to standard care and no treatment.
Ref. 5	RCT	Individual traditional Chinese AC and moxibustion vs sham	28	8 sessions 4 weeks	Symptom severity/improvement. Clinical Global Impression Scale	Statistically significant improvement in pain, gas, bloating, and stool consistency in control group
Ref. 10	Pilot study Pragmatic RCT	AC with usual care vs usual care alone	30	10 sessions	IBS-SSS at 3 months	More research into AC for IBS merited
Ref. 3	RCT Longitudinal evaluation	Standard vs np-SAC at non-AP points	22 AC; 21 np-SAC	10 sessions 5 weeks	QOL	Increased QOL in both groups. No significant difference between groups.
Ref. 8	RCT Longitudinal evaluation	Individual AC vs p-SAC	27 AC; 32 p-SAC	10 sessions 10 weeks	Symptom score Quality of life	Improved in both groups. No significant difference between groups.

(continued)

Table 44-1 Continued
Clinical Trials of Acupuncture in IBS

Ref. 11	RCT with cross-over design. Longitudinal evaluation.	Electro-AC vs np-SAC on AC points	9 IBS; 12 health	2 treatment (1) AC (1) PAC	Perception threshold with barostat	Increased in both groups. No significant difference between groups.
Ref. 12	Cross-over trial. Cross-sectional and longitudinal evaluation.	TENS vs Sham TENS	24 IBS-D; 20 IBS-C; 30 CC; 30 health	8 treatments 2 months	Perception threshold with barostat	Increased in IBS-D. Significant group difference.
Ref. 7	Cross-over design. Longitudinal evaluation.	AC at LI 4 vs p-AC at BL 60	25	4 treatments 4 weeks	Symptoms	Improved in both groups after first treatment with P=0.05 for AC. No significant difference between groups after second treatment.
Ref. 6	Pilot study	No control	7	4 weeks	Symptom scores	Acupuncture effective (P<0.01)
Ref. 9	RCT	Psychotherapy vs AC vs p-SAC vs papaverine vs placebo	60	Unclear	Subjective symptom scores	Psychotherapy superior to AC and papaverine (P<0.01). AC superior to p-SAC (P<0.01).

Adapted from Schneider A, Enck P, Streitberger K, et al. Acupuncture treatment in irritable bowel syndrome. *Gut.* 2006;55:649-654.

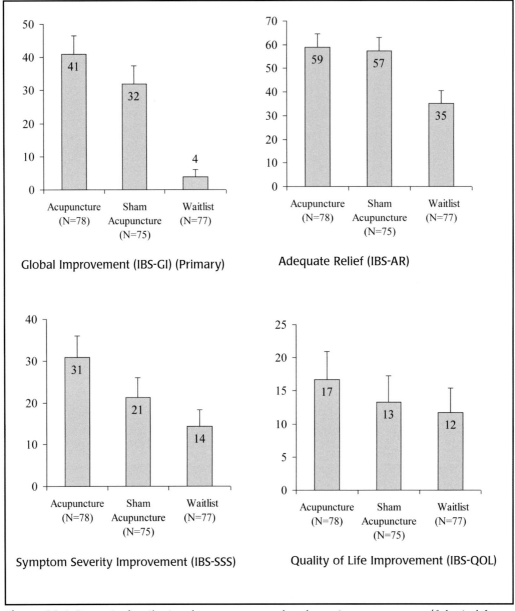

Figure 44-1. Percent of patients who were responders by outcome measure. (Adapted from Lembo AJ, Conboy L, Kelley JM, et al. A treatment trial of acupuncture in IBS patients. *Am J Gastroenterol.* 2009;104:1489-1497).

study by Lembo and colleagues,[4] 230 IBS patients were randomized to 6 acupuncture treatment sessions using 6 fixed and 11 optional (ie, based on a traditional Chinese acupuncture diagnosis) acupoints following a 3-week "run-in" with sham acupuncture in an "augmented" or "limited" patient-practitioner interaction. A third arm of the study included a wait-list control group. There was a non-statistically significant improvement in most of the IBS global endpoints between acupuncture and sham acupuncture (Figure 44-1). However, there was a significant improvement in IBS global endpoints between acupuncture and sham acupuncture, and wait-list control.

While it is not clear on the basis of published literature that acupuncture will help the majority of patients with IBS, it is unlikely to cause harm, appears to be superior to no treatment or standard IBS treatment, and may result in improvement of symptoms in some patients. We recommend acupuncture for those patients with IBS with persistent symptoms of pain who are either interested in and receptive to alternative therapies or who have failed traditional therapies. However, one of the difficulties with acupuncture is finding a provider who is skilled and knowledgeable in the treatment of patients with functional bowel disorders.

References

1. Lim B, Manheimer E, Lao L, et al. Acupuncture for treatment of irritable bowel syndrome. *Cochrane Database Syst Rev*. 2006:CD005111.
2. Schneider A, Streitberger K, Joos S. Acupuncture treatment in gastrointestinal diseases: a systematic review. *World J Gastroenterol*. 2007;13:3417-3424.
3. Schneider A, Enck P, Streitberger K, et al. Acupuncture treatment in irritable bowel syndrome. *Gut*. 2006;55:649-654.
4. Lembo AJ, Conboy L, Kelley JM, et al. A treatment trial of acupuncture in IBS patients. *Am J Gastroenterol*. 2009;104:1489-1497.
5. Anastasi JK, McMahon DJ, Kim GH. Symptom management for irritable bowel syndrome: a pilot randomized controlled trial of acupuncture/moxibustion. *Gastroenterol Nurs*. 2009;32:243-255.
6. Chan J, Carr I, Mayberry JF. The role of acupuncture in the treatment of irritable bowel syndrome: a pilot study. *Hepatogastroenterology*. 1997;44:1328-1330.
7. Fireman Z, Segal A, Kopelman Y, Sternberg A, Carasso R. Acupuncture treatment for irritable bowel syndrome. A double-blind controlled study. *Digestion*. 2001;64:100-103.
8. Forbes A, Jackson S, Walter C, Quraishi S, Jacyna M, Pitcher M. Acupuncture for irritable bowel syndrome: a blinded placebo-controlled trial. *World J Gastroenterol*. 2005;11:4040-4044.
9. Kunze M, Seidel HJ, Stube G. Comparative studies of the effectiveness of brief psychotherapy, acupuncture and papaverin therapy in patients with irritable bowel syndrome. *Z Gesamte Inn Med*. 1990;45:625-627.
10. Reynolds JA, Bland JM, MacPherson H. Acupuncture for irritable bowel syndrome an exploratory randomised controlled trial. *Acupunct Med*. 2008;26:8-16.
11. Rohrbock RB, Hammer J, Vogelsang H, Talley NJ, Hammer HF. Acupuncture has a placebo effect on rectal perception but not on distensibility and spatial summation: a study in health and IBS. *Am J Gastroenterol*. 2004;99:1990-1997.
12. Xiao WB, Liu YL. Rectal hypersensitivity reduced by acupoint TENS in patients with diarrhea-predominant irritable bowel syndrome: a pilot study. *Dig Dis Sci*. 2004;49:312-319.
13. Lim B, Manheimer E, Lao L. Acupuncture treatment of IBS. *Cochrane Database Syst Rev*. 2006;CD005111.

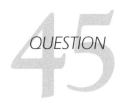
WILL HYPNOTHERAPY HELP
MY PATIENTS WITH IBS?

Basma Issa, MD, MPhil and
Peter Whorwell, BSc, MB, BS, MD, PhD, FRCP

It is well-known that there is tremendous variation in the severity of irritable bowel syndrome (IBS) symptoms, with many patients experiencing only relatively mild symptoms on an infrequent basis. However, at the other end of the spectrum, there are patients in whom the condition is much more severe with the potential to completely ruin their lives. In this group of patients, symptoms tend to be continuous with pain often being a predominant feature. Patients may also experience extremes of bowel dysfunction characterized by very infrequent bowel movements or diarrhea, the latter of which may be associated with urgency and incontinence. Typically, these individuals also suffer from a variety of "noncolonic" symptoms including lethargy, low backache, nausea, and a range of urinary as well gynecologic symptoms. Even though such patients represent a minority of the totality of IBS patients because the condition is so common, they are still relatively numerous. Not surprisingly, these severely affected patients are challenging to treat, partly because their symptoms are so intense but also because their symptoms are so diverse; it is thus difficult to conceive of a pharmacological approach that might help all of them. The tricyclic antidepressants are the pharmacologic agents that possibly come closest to achieving this goal, but even these compounds only have a finite success rate. As a referral center, we see large numbers of such cases of severe IBS where treatment has been unsuccessful and the sufferer is becoming increasingly despondent about the prospects of any help in the future, especially as they have often been told "there is nothing more that can be done for you." It is in this group that we consider the possibility of trying hypnotherapy.

Unfortunately, hypnotherapy is very time consuming, as well as costly to provide, and even in our unit with five therapists, it can be associated with a long waiting list. Consequently, it is important to establish that the patient is truly refractory to medical and dietary therapy before embarking on a course of hypnotherapy. We, therefore, re-visit all of their previous medications, especially antidepressants, to ensure that they have been used at adequate doses for adequate periods of time, and we pay particular attention to their diet where we often achieve surprisingly good results with somewhat unconventional manipulations. Even small improvements at this stage are worthwhile, as any reduction in symptoms means there is less for hypnotherapy to overcome. Patients often view hypnosis as their last hope of salvation and not surprisingly become very distressed if they fail to respond to this form of treatment. Consequently, it is essential to have a strategy for dealing with these individuals, which in our unit takes the form of at least providing continuing support and care, but also acknowledging the fact that any further improvement is rather unlikely.

The hypnotherapy that we provide is called "gut focused hypnosis." This is based on the premise that hypnosis can enable the subject to modify physiological functions not immediately accessible to conscious control, and we and others have accumulated evidence that this hypothesis is true in relation to the gastrointestinal system.[1] Thus, the patient with IBS is taught strategies to try and control the various putative pathophysiological abnormalities that are thought to contribute to their condition in order to bring about symptom relief. We make absolutely no attempt to deal with or explore any deep-seated psychological or traumatic issues as we are a gastrointestinal unit and are not equipped to cross that boundary. However, it goes without saying that hypnosis is good for stress and anxiety, and we are perfectly happy to address this aspect of their problem. It therefore appears that hypnosis offers control of a wide range of parameters, and this might explain why it helps the whole symptom profile of the patient. Not only do the traditional symptoms of IBS improve, but so do all the "noncolonic" symptoms, as well as features such as anxiety and depression. This is in stark contrast to pharmacological approaches, which often only help the abdominal pain or the bowel dysfunction depending on the drug and hardly ever help features such as lethargy or low backache.

Following our original controlled trial in 1984 demonstrating the efficacy of hypnotherapy in IBS, we have been continuously providing this form of treatment for sufferers, and despite the increasingly severe nature of the cases being sent to us these days, we still manage to achieve a success rate of approximately 70%. Obviously, this figure depends on how you define success, and for the purposes of audit and publication, we consider treatment has been successful if a patient says that compared with before treatment, his or her symptoms have been reduced by 50% or more.[2,3] It is vital that the individual understands that IBS, just like conditions such as migraine or asthma, is not curable but we can teach them to control the condition. Furthermore, offering such a form of treatment would not make sense unless the beneficial effects were sustained and we have confirmed that the majority of successfully treated individuals remain well up to and beyond 5 years.

A response rate of 70% means that 30 out of every 100 patients we treat fail to gain benefit from this modality, and it would be nice if we could predict responders to save the others the consequences of treatment failure, which can be emotionally quite traumatic. To date, we have not really been successful in this quest, although there are some common sense observations that can be made in the clinic, of which noting the patient's attitude is probably the best predictor of response. Healthy skepticism is not a problem but if there is a belief in a particular individual that this particular form of treatment is not going to work then it is probably not even worth trying. Patients need to know that they are learning a skill, and it is essential that they participate fully in the treatment process and practice the technique, preferably on a daily basis, at least during the active treatment phase.

In contrast to the usual doctor-patient interaction where patients are given a medication and passively wait for it to work, in our hypnotherapy unit, they are taught an active skill that they then have to make work for themselves. Although we have never tried hypnotherapy in mild patients, we feel it may not be successful in this group, as there may not be sufficient motivation to practice enough to reach an adequate skill level. More recently, we have been assessing response to hypnotherapy in relation to the patients' imagery of their disease as well as how they perceive colors, and some interesting results are beginning to emerge. However, these data are far too preliminary for clinical application.

The success of our IBS hypnotherapy program has encouraged us to explore its utility in other functional gastrointestinal disorders, and we now have positive evidence in support of its use in functional dyspepsia as well as noncardiac chest pain. In addition, we have some preliminary data suggesting that it may even be helpful in inflammatory bowel disease, and this and all the other research we have undertaken over the years is covered in detail in the review cited below.

References

1. Miller V, Whorwell PJ. Hypnotherapy for functional gastrointestinal disorders: a review. *Int J Clin Exp Hypn.* 2009;57(3):279-292.
2. Gonsalkorale WM, Houghton LA, Whorwell PJ. Hypnotherapy in irritable bowel syndrome: a large-scale audit of a clinical service with examination of factors influencing responsiveness. *Am J Gastroenterol.* 2002;97(4):954-961.
3. Gonsalkorale WM, Miller V, Afzal A, Whorwell PJ. Long term benefits of hypnotherapy for irritable bowel syndrome. *Gut.* 2003;52(11):1623-1629.

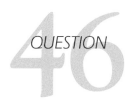

WHAT IS BEHAVIORAL THERAPY AND WILL IT HELP MY PATIENTS WITH IBS?

Chris Radziwon, PhD and Jeff Lackner, PsyD

The past 20 years has witnessed the development and application of multiple psychosocial therapies for irritable bowel syndrome (IBS). Their theoretical roots are grounded in the biopsychosocial model that holds that individual biology (eg, genetic predisposition, GI physiology), behavior, and higher-order cognitive processes (coping, illness beliefs, abnormal central processing of gut stimuli) influence the expression of IBS symptoms through their interaction with each other, with early life factors (eg, trauma, modeling, parenting practices), and with the individual's sociocultural environment (eg, reinforcement contingencies). Research based on the biopsychosocial model points to three main pathways through which psychological factors are believed to influence IBS. The first pathway is directly through biological systems that mediate gut function and sensation. The second pathway is through the adoption of illness behaviors that exacerbate IBS symptoms, obscure symptom profile, and compromise function. Health behaviors are strongly influenced by psychosocial factors.[1] A third pathway is by mediating the risk for development of chronic IBS symptoms, which usually involves focusing on the high rates of early life adversity in patients seeking treatment. To the extent that psychological factors influence the expression of IBS, it is believed that symptoms are more effectively managed by addressing their presumed underlying psychosocial processes. By targeting one of the pathways linking psychological factors to IBS, psychological treatments presumably cause an improvement in symptoms or other outcome parameters (eg, function, healthcare use, quality of life).

Of different psychotherapies targeted for IBS, cognitive behavioral therapy (CBT) is the most widely studied and empirically validated.[1] CBT is a brief, highly structured, problem-focused, and prescriptive therapy based on 3 central underlying assumptions:

1. Patients have specific skills deficits that render them vulnerable to symptom exacerbations
2. Formal instruction in skills for modifying (unlearning) maladaptive behaviors and thinking patterns remediate (learning) skills deficits
3. Remediation of skills deficits stands to promote symptom relief.

In CBT, treatment involves a detailed, ongoing assessment of a patient's problems. This assessment focuses on the immediate (versus historical) determinants of the problem for which the patient seeks relief. The assumption is that, at a clinical level, individuals are best characterized by what they think, feel, and do in specific situations. This information provides an understanding of how clinical problems are maintained and what treatment techniques should be deployed to tackle different facets of a given problem. Because CBT is based on the principles and procedures of experimental psychology, behavioral treatment methods are precisely specified and based on the results of controlled clinical research, not clinical intuition or anecdote. In our clinical practice and through our National Institutes of Health (NIH)-funded research, we have emphasized more cognitively oriented interventions such as cognitive restructuring, problem-solving, and self-monitoring of symptoms, their antecedents and consequences. This approach reflects the apparent limited incremental benefit of noncognitive interventions, such as biofeedback, as stand-alone procedures and the important role of central processes on the neuroenteric axis.

Cognitive restructuring techniques are designed to challenge and dispute negatively skewed thinking patterns characteristic of patients with IBS. These techniques are based on the assumption that cognitive processes (ie, patients' perceptions, attributions, and beliefs) reflect errors and biases in the way they process information and can influence symptom exacerbations. Our work focuses on patients' perceptions of uncontrollability and unpredictability because they moderate the experience of excessive stress that many IBS patients link to flare-ups of GI symptoms.[2,3] People who experience excessive stress perceive themselves to be at the mercy of unpredictable demands on their resources and/or are unable to control these demands even if they are able to predict them. This cognitive style is reflected in intense (ie, excessive and uncontrollable) worry. A tendency to worry is regarded as an attempt to predict future negative events and is manifested in very discrete patterns of thinking: tendencies to catastrophize (overestimate the cost or consequences of negative events), to overestimate the likelihood of threat (thinking the worst), and to exaggerate the controllability of events. An IBS patient may be reluctant to travel on a plane because of worries she will lose control of her bowels and embarrass herself in front of other passengers. In this case, the patient overestimates how likely the anticipated negative event will occur, and such risk inflation triggers both anxiety and IBS symptoms.

To the extent that patients can link catastrophic cognitions to symptom flare-ups using daily symptom records, they would be encouraged to test the validity and usefulness of negative thoughts and their impact on symptoms. Patients are instructed to challenge and dispute negatively skewed thinking patterns using a variety of techniques. One common strategy requires the patient to learn and apply evidence-based logic ("what is the probability that my worry of having an accident on the plane will definitely occur based on the evidence I have right now") to generate more factual predictions ("I really don't know what's going to happen…while I had one accident several years ago, the majority of plane trips have not been a problem") rather than threatening interpretations of life events. By rehearsing structured exercises between clinic visits, patients learn to identify problem beliefs, challenge and dispute their accuracy, and reduce the intensity of responses.

As patients grow more proficient in challenging IBS-related automatic thoughts, the cognitive restructuring component of CBT shifts to modifying dysfunctional assumptions or "core beliefs." Core beliefs are global, deeply ingrained assumptions individuals hold regarding the world. Core beliefs such as perfectionism ("If I do something, it has to be flawless or its junk") and expectation of approval ("If other people do not like me all the time, then I am worthless") are believed to trigger automatic thoughts that underlie maladaptive response patterns.

Another cognitive intervention is flexible problem-solving training. Problem-solving training is a systematic approach to dealing with problems emphasizing five stages of information processing (defining the problem, generating alternative solutions, weighting their relative value and costs, decision making, and verification). Our focus is on teaching patients a flexible problem-solving approach that helps them manage both controllable and uncontrollable problems. This clinical approach emanates from behavioral medicine research showing that patients with functional GI disorders tend to rely on action-oriented problem-solving responses that are geared toward fixing or solving a problem regardless of the "true" controllability of a stressor. Their overreliance on action-oriented approaches reflects a tendency to rigidly appraise problems as controllable. Therefore, we teach patients to make accurate estimations of the controllability of a stressor and then apply an appropriate problem-solving approach. For uncontrollable problems, patients are taught to use strategies geared toward managing the emotional unpleasantness of the situation (eg, acceptance/resignation, "letting go," reinterpretation). For controllable stressors, patients are taught to use strategies that are geared toward solving or "fixing" the situation itself.

In our clinical research program at the University at Buffalo,[2] we also teach patients muscle relaxation strategies to dampen heightened physiological arousal and increase a sense of mastery over symptoms. We typically emphasize either progressive muscle relaxation training or diaphragmatic breathing. Progressive muscle relaxation training consists of the systematic tensing and relaxing of selected muscle groups of the whole body. Tension release cycles are used to deepen relaxation and to sharpen the patient's ability to detect tension sooner after it develops. The patient first learns to achieve deep relaxation with a relatively lengthy 16 muscle group tension-relaxation exercise. Once patients master 16 muscle group exercises, they learn skills to achieve physical relaxation with fewer muscle groups until they can elicit a relaxation response without tensing any muscles. It is believed that unless patients detect tension early and respond to it more adaptively (by applying a more adaptive coping response), physical tension may accumulate to a point that it aggravates or amplifies body systems. Another relaxation skill is breathing retraining. In breathing retraining, the patient is taught to take slow, deep, even abdominal/diaphragmatic breaths and to attend to relaxing sensations during exhalation. Breathing patterns (eg, shallow, chest breathing), if chronic, can intensify physiological arousal that underlies somatic symptoms aggravated by stress. By learning to slow down respiration through diaphragmatic breathing, patients presumably reduce the intensity of physical symptoms. As with all CBT strategies, breathing retraining requires patients to carry out daily practice exercises between sessions to facilitate skills acquisition and generalize skills taught in the clinic to the home setting.

CBT techniques discussed have been administered either singly (eg, cognitive restructuring or relaxation techniques alone as treatments) or in combination with other interventions and have been featured in 24 randomized clinical trials since 1985. The first generation of CBT trials suffered from many methodological flaws. However, as the quality of trials has improved, a clearer picture of CBT's therapeutic value has emerged. In comparison with passive control conditions (eg, wait list, no-treatment, treatment as usual), CBT generally yields broad improvements in GI symptoms (pain, bowel dysfunction) and quality of life. Interestingly, CBT appears more effective in reducing GI symptoms than coexisting psychological ones such as anxiety or depression.[3] Research summarized in a recent meta-analysis suggests that psychological treatments as a whole are at least moderately effective in reducing core symptoms of IBS (ie, abdominal pain, problem bowel habits). Although there were not enough data to establish the relative superiority of any one type of psychological treatment, 14 of 17 trials in the meta-analysis featured CBT. A recent study[4] using CBT to treat severely affected IBS patients found that the great majority of patients reported significant reduction in the severity of IBS symptoms and reported adequate relief from IBS symptoms.[4] Another important finding of this study was that CBT's most robust effect was on gastrointestinal symptoms, not psychological distress. The therapeutic value of CBT was echoed in a recently published *New England Journal of Medicine* narrative review[5] that identified CBT as one of the few empirically validated treatments for IBS and is the only treatment—dietary, pharmacological, or behavioral, found to be efficacious for the full range of IBS symptoms.

References

1. Levy RL, Olden KW, Naliboff BD, et al. Psychosocial aspects of the functional gastrointestinal disorders. *Gastroenterology.* 2006;130(5):1447-1458.
2. Lackner JM. *Controlling IBS the Drug-Free Way: A 10-Step Plan for Symptom Relief.* New York: Stewart, Tabori, & Chang; 2008.
3. Lackner JM, Mesmer C, Morley S, Dowzer C, Hamilton S. Psychological treatments for irritable bowel syndrome: a systematic review and meta-analysis. *J Consult Clin Psychol.* 2004;72(6):1100-1113.
4. Lackner JM, Jaccard J, Krasner SS, Katz LA, Gudleski GD, Holroyd K. Self-administered cognitive behavior therapy for moderate to severe irritable bowel syndrome: clinical efficacy, tolerability, feasability. *Clinical Gastroenterology Hepatology.* 2008;6(8):899-906.
5. Mayer EA. Clinical practice. Irritable bowel syndrome. *N Engl J Med.* 2008;358(16):1692-1699.

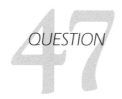
IBS AND CAM: WHAT OPTIONS ARE AVAILABLE?

Richard Nahas, MD, CCFP

It is important for physicians who treat patients with irritable bowel syndrome (IBS) to know about complementary and alternative medicine (CAM). Almost one-half of IBS patients report using CAM. In many patients, this is because their symptoms have not been adequately treated by standard approaches. Others report turning to CAM because their physicians do not take their complaints seriously or because they feel they have not received a thorough evaluation. For a variety of reasons, many IBS patients who use CAM therapies do not tell their doctor.

The diagnosis of IBS is made in patients with specific symptoms whose clinical evaluation does not reveal organic pathology (see Chapter 4). While the symptoms are generally consistent, most CAM practitioners, including physicians and nonmedical practitioners, consider IBS to be a state of dysfunction with a number of potential contributing factors. As such, the treatment of IBS from a CAM perspective seeks to identify and correct these contributing factors in addition to treating the symptoms of dysfunction.

Treating Symptoms

A more detailed review of the CAM therapies discussed here was recently published.[1] The physiologic abnormality that has been most consistently described in patients with IBS in the medical literature is visceral hypersensitivity. As such, the most obvious approach includes therapies that address the mind-brain-gut axis. Serotonergic agents target this axis, but many mind-body medicine modalities lend themselves well to this therapeutic strategy, particularly among patients who report that their symptoms are worse when they are under psychological stress or emotional strain.

Clinical hypnosis involves helping patients achieve a state of deep relaxation and narrow focus, during which therapeutic suggestions are made. Gut-directed hypnotherapy is a specific technique that combines suggestions related to emotional well-being and intestinal health. A Cochrane review of 4 hypnotherapy trials in 147 patients with

IBS reported positive outcomes in all trials, although methodologic issues make these findings inconclusive (see Chapter 45).

Cognitive behavioral therapy (CBT) is a form of counseling that trains patients to recognize thoughts and behaviors that amplify symptoms or undermine well-being and replace them with healthier ones. The largest trial of individual CBT included 431 patients who received 12 weekly sessions of CBT or an educational program. The response rate was 70% in the CBT group versus 37% in the active control group ($P<0.001$). Other small trials of individual and group CBT yielded similarly promising results (see Chapter 46).

Other mind-body techniques may be more readily available, and many patients will be more likely to try an intervention that is simple and easy to do. Patient education CDs that teach progressive muscle relaxation, guided imagery, breathing techniques, and other mind-body practices are available at bookstores or online. While no single intervention has been rigorously studied, many of our patients have reported significant benefit after 1 to 2 weeks of use. Their low cost, safety, and ease of use make them worth considering.

Many herbal preparations have been used to treat IBS, one of which is **peppermint oil**. An extract of *Mentha piperita* relaxes intestinal smooth muscle via its calcium channel-blocking effect, and 2 meta-analyses have demonstrated a consistent reduction in abdominal pain in patients who used 3 to 6 capsules per day. They are enteric-coated to prevent heartburn, as peppermint can cause lower esophageal sphincter relaxation. Reported side effects include nausea and mild perianal burning.

Asian **herbal formulas** have also been tested in randomized trials. These include a traditional Chinese medicine formula called tong xie yao fang and a Tibetan formula known as Padma Lax. Trials have also been conducted on a European formula named STW 5 and another named Iberogast. The latter formula has been shown to be effective in functional dyspepsia. Large, randomized, placebo-controlled trials are lacking in IBS.

Probiotic bacteria, including *Lactobacillus* and *Bifidobacter* species, can be very effective in some patients. Their use was popularized in the late 19th century by Nobel laureate Elie Metchnikoff, who linked the health of Balkan peasants to their consumption of kefir, a fermented milk drink. Other probiotic-rich fermented foods include kefir, miso, tempeh, and sauerkraut. These bacteria produce short-chain fatty acids, deconjugate bile acids, limit the growth of pathogenic bacteria, and interact with gut-associated lymphoid tissue to promote immune tolerance and attenuate visceral hypersensitivity. A meta-analysis of 23 trials involving 1404 patients found improvement in abdominal pain and global IBS symptoms.[2] Daily oral doses of 10 to 100 billion bacteria are most commonly used. There is no clear evidence favoring one particular type of probiotic, but most products include several strains (see Chapters 41 and 42).

Finding the Underlying Cause

As mentioned above, many CAM providers consider IBS to be a descriptive diagnosis representing a state of dysfunction that can be related to a number of potential contributing factors. These are often revealed by clues in the clinical history that may require detailed questioning to uncover.

Patients who report extensive **travel** in developing countries may harbor parasites that are often missed by conventional stool testing, and empiric treatment may be considered.

Some patients may have symptoms related to nonsteroidal anti-inflammatory drugs, beta-blockers, or other **medication** use. Patients who report lifelong abdominal symptoms should be asked about **feeding during infancy**. Many find out from their parents that they developed severe colic when breastfeeding was stopped. This would suggest a problem with lactose or casein that may require a brief dairy-free trial to identify. A significant number of patients develop IBS symptoms shortly after an episode of **gastroenteritis**, and in some patients they begin after receiving an **antibiotic**. This may lead the clinician to suspect small intestinal bacterial overgrowth (flora in the wrong place) or increased intestinal permeability (leaky gut syndrome), both of which are readily diagnosed using standardized tests. Probiotics would be more helpful in these patients.

A more controversial hypothesis is that these acute insults can temporarily alter gut flora and immune function, leading to the development of new **food allergies**. While skin IgE testing may reveal food allergy, this test for type 1 hypersensitivity is best suited to identifying environmental allergens. Other allergy testing, including serum IgG antibody panels and electrodermal and applied kinesiology tests, are unproven and are not generally recommended. In our experience, they can be unreliable, although some patients have found them very useful. Interestingly, in a double-blind trial of IgG food antibody testing in IBS patients, those who eliminated allergens from a "real" test improved more than those who eliminated foods based on a "sham" test.[3] The "gold standard" is an **elimination diet** that begins with 3 to 4 simple foods (eg, water, chicken broth, boiled chicken, white rice) for a week and then introduces 1 new food ingredient every 1 to 2 days. This is clinically useful but can be arduous, so patients should be advised to consult a nutritionist or dietician for help. The recommended treatment is avoidance.

Gluten sensitivity is a particularly contentious issue among IBS patients and their physicians. Many CAM providers report very positive results in biopsy-negative patients who have undergone a gluten-free trial. These patients often report that their symptoms dramatically improve or disappear after 1 to 2 months, and they also report clear symptoms when they eat gluten. These re-exposures are often accidental and unknown to the patient until after they develop symptoms and retrace their steps to uncover the offending gluten-containing food. It is important to state that this phenomenon has not been reported in the medical literature, but there is a veritable explosion of interest in this issue in IBS patients and society-at-large, so studies confirming or refuting it are urgently needed.

The treatment of IBS is a good example of the importance of integrative medicine. This approach combines conventional medical diagnosis and treatment with safe, effective CAM therapies, emphasizes the patient instead of the disease, and is based on an understanding of how different body systems interact and influence each other. The relationship between the gastrointestinal system, the nervous system, and the immune system often plays a role in the development of IBS and can help guide treatment. Physicians should ask patients about their use of CAM therapies and providers and should listen respectfully to their thoughts and feelings to establish a therapeutic alliance. Many CAM approaches can be recommended based on the comfort level of the physician, or patients can be referred to a naturopathic doctor or integrative medical doctor if one is available.

References

1. Shen YA, Nahas R. Complementary and alternative medicine for treatment of irritable bowel syndrome. *Can Fam Phys.* 2009;55:143-148.

2. McFarland LV, Dublin S. Meta-analysis of probiotics for the treatment of irritable bowel syndrome. *World J Gastroenterol.* 2008;14:2650-2661.
3. Atkinson W, Sheldon TA, Shaath N, Whorwell PJ. Food elimination based on IgG antibodies in irritable bowel syndrome: a randomized controlled trial. *Gut.* 2004;53:1459-1464.

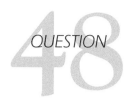
WHAT IS THE BEST APPROACH FOR TREATING ABDOMINAL PAIN IN PATIENTS WITH IBS?

Madhusudan Grover, MD and Douglas A. Drossman, MD

Irritable bowel syndrome (IBS) is characterized by the presence of recurrent abdominal pain or discomfort associated with defecation or a change in bowel habit and with features of disordered defecation. Table 48-1 lists the Rome III diagnostic criteria for the diagnosis of IBS. The Rome III classification also differentiates IBS from nonpainful disorders of defecation (ie, functional diarrhea or functional constipation) and from abdominal pain not associated with problems of defecation (eg, functional abdominal pain syndrome).[1] Irritable bowel syndrome is not the most common functional gastrointestinal disorder (FGID), but it is certainly the most extensively studied one. On survey analysis, up to 7% to 20% of adults fulfill the diagnostic criteria for IBS; however, most of these do not seek health care. Despite this, approximately 2% of adult primary-care visits and up to one-half of primary gastroenterologists' visits can be from IBS patients. These patients are often subjected to expensive investigations ("to rule out an organic pathology"), hospitalization, and unwarranted abdominal and gynecological surgeries. The direct and indirect medical costs for IBS amount to approximately $20 to $30 billion dollars annually in the United States.

Abdominal Pain in IBS

Even though "pain" associated with bowel dysfunction is the characteristic feature of IBS, there has been limited research looking specifically at targeting the pain. Pain can be a feature of both IBS with diarrhea (IBS-D) and IBS with constipation (IBS-C). The diagnosis of IBS usually remains stable over time. However, patients may move from one subtype (eg, either IBS-D or IBS-C) to another over time (eg, alternating symptoms of

---

Table 48-1
Rome III Criteria for Diagnosis of IBS*

Recurrent abdominal pain or discomfort** at least 3 days/month in the past 3 months associated with 2 or more of the following:
- Improvement with defecation
- Onset associated with a change in frequency of stool
- Onset associated with a change in form (appearance) of stool

*Criterion fulfilled for the past 3 months with symptom onset at least 6 months prior to diagnosis.
**"Discomfort" means an uncomfortable sensation not described as pain.

---

constipation and diarrhea, IBS-A). Generally, the severity of IBS seems to correlate with the severity of pain rather than the severity of bowel symptoms (ie, diarrhea or constipation).[2] Severity also creates a spectrum of patients ranging from patients in the community not seeking health care to patients in primary care or primary GI practice to patients seen at tertiary referral centers. The more severe patients tend to have poorer quality of life, work absenteeism, frequent healthcare seeking, and more psychosocial distress.

Evaluating Pain in IBS

There has been a gradual shift in the process of making the diagnosis of IBS and other FGIDs from a "negative diagnosis (ie, diagnosis of exclusion)" to a "positive diagnosis (fulfillment of Rome criteria)" approach. In the absence of red flags (see Table 48-2), a confident positive diagnosis of IBS enhances patient confidence and facilitates development of a therapeutic doctor-patient relationship. It also saves the physician time and energy and allows the physician to focus on managing the symptoms rather than embarking on an exhaustive process of ruling out several "organic" diagnoses first, which is often expensive and of low yield.

From a clinical practice standpoint, imagine a 30-year-old woman in your office with diarrhea-predominant symptoms who fulfills symptom criteria as listed in Table 48-1 and does not have any of the alarm symptoms listed in Table 48-2. What are the chances of uncovering an alternate diagnosis after pursuing additional work-up? Recent studies suggest that the likelihood is very small. In fact, a study has shown a lower prevalence of colorectal adenomas in patients with "suspected" nonconstipated IBS as compared to controls. Thus, we do not advise pursuing additional and often repetitive diagnostic tests when a positive diagnosis of IBS can be established from the symptoms and no red flags/alarm symptoms are present.

We think that in patients with chronic abdominal pain, such as in IBS, important information can be obtained from a detailed psychosocial history (Table 48-3). We try to obtain a "snapshot" life history of the illness within a psychosocial context and attempt

---

Table 48-2

Red Flags During Evaluating Patient With Suspected IBS

- Blood in stool
- Awakened by GI symptoms
- Unintended weight loss
- Family history of colon cancer or IBD
- Symptom onset after age 50

Table 48-3

Psychosocial Assessment in Evaluation of Pain in IBS

1. Life history of illness
   Evaluate if acute vs chronic and the presence of other chronic pain conditions.
2. Reasons for seeking care now
   Associated concerns, triggers, worsening functional and/or psychosocial status.
3. Life history of traumatic events
   Access history of abuse, personal or family losses.
4. Patient's understanding of illness
   Recognizing mind-body interactions vs looking for an organic cause.
5. Impact of pain on activities and quality of life
   To plan diagnostic and treatment decisions
6. Associated psychiatric diagnosis
   Diagnose and treat Axis I and Axis II psychiatric disorders.
7. Role of family and culture
   Recognize dysfunctional family interactions and cultural belief systems.
8. Associated psychosocial impairment and available resources
   Help seek social networks and avoid maladaptive coping (catastrophizing).

---

to understand life history factors that may have contributed to pain origin and exacerbations. Following that, the reasons for seeking care should be assessed looking for specific fears (eg, loss of a close friend or relative with similar symptoms, abuse, etc). We should try to assess their understanding of illness ("What do you think is causing this?"). Factors that affect them the most ("Of all of these symptoms, what worries you the most?") and their fears ("What do you think will happen if these symptoms do not go away?") can help provide further insight into a complex set of symptoms and can help plan treatment. Ultimately, understanding these factors to the best degree possible fosters development of a therapeutic relationship with our patients.

Managing Pain in IBS

GENERAL PRINCIPLES

Pain associated with IBS is usually managed according to severity and can differ significantly between a primary/general GI practice and a tertiary-care referral center where very different patient populations can be encountered. However, the process of care begins with validating the patients' symptoms and explaining the pathophysiological basis for them. We find that drawing figures to explain brain-gut interactions can be extremely useful. Fear of cancer is very common in IBS patients seen in primary care, and reassurance is often infrequent but can be very therapeutic. Repeated investigations may reflect physician uncertainty and can feed into patient anxiety and fear, thus perpetuating a cycle of ineffective management.

SETTING AGENDA

Patients with IBS can feel helpless in the presence of their symptoms and thus may prefer not to take responsibility for symptom management. Physicians may feel burdened by this imposed expectation and can display attitudes that are not conducive to a therapeutic relationship. We find that the best approach is to communicate willingness to work on the symptoms with the patient in a collaborative fashion—one in which the patient is encouraged to take a greater role in the decision making. This helps patients regain their sense of control. At the same time, it is important to set treatment goals and clearly discuss expectations in terms of your time, follow-up appointments, and returning phone calls. Studies have shown that patient recall of the diagnosis and understanding and recollection of the management plan can be poor after any one office visit. This makes it important to continue to see the patient in follow-up so that a deeper understanding of the disorder and its treatments can be reinforced. It also reassures them and increases patients' confidence in your willingness to work on their symptoms. Table 48-4 lists some of the general principles of managing pain in IBS.

DIET

Patients most commonly believe that food types and other dietary factors are the primary causes for their symptoms. In part, this may relate to the personal experience of symptoms occurring in relation to eating, information received from family and friends, and the need to achieve some meaning in their symptom experiences in order to have a sense of control ("effort after meaning"). Nevertheless, the knowledge of the role of these factors needs to be placed in a proper clinical context. For example, patients may avoid eating selected foods due to the fact that they experience symptoms when eating. But this may relate more to filling the stomach (distention) and the release of various neuropeptides rather than to the particular type of food eaten. Thus, elimination diets may not always be helpful. Also, there is a poor correlation between reported lactose intolerance and true lactose malabsorption. Celiac disease can mimic many symptoms of IBS and should be included in the differential diagnosis. We find that daily food diaries can be useful in recognizing patterns of dietary triggers before implementing any food elimina-

---

Table 48-4

General Treatment Principles for Managing Pain in IBS

Establishing an effective patient-physician relationship
1. Empathy
2. Education
3. Validation
4. Reassurance
5. Negotiate the treatment
6. Set reasonable limits

The treatment plan:
1. Set reasonable treatment goals
2. Help the patient take responsibility
3. Base treatment on symptom severity and the degree of disability
4. Medications
5. Mental health referral
6. Specific psychological treatments
7. Multidisciplinary pain treatment center referral

---

tion. For example, lactose elimination without evidence of lactose intolerance producing symptoms can deplete a useful dietary source of calcium, and gluten restriction without evidence for gluten intolerance can be expensive and difficult to maintain. However, if no patterns are seen and if discomfort is mostly associated with bloating, a trial of lactose elimination can be useful, especially in populations with a high incidence of lactose intolerance such as Asians and African Americans. Occasionally, a trial of fructose elimination can be useful, and avoidance of complex polysaccharides (FODMAPS) should be considered (see Chapter 30).

GUT ACTING MEDICATIONS

The treatment of abdominal pain associated with milder/infrequent symptoms is usually accomplished by managing their bowel symptoms (eg, treating the symptoms of diarrhea or constipation). For example, many patients with mild symptoms of IBS with diarrhea note an improvement in their abdominal pain when treated with smooth-muscle relaxants (eg, dicyclomine, hyoscyamine). However, there is little evidence to support their use when the abdominal pain is more severe or when it is not related to meals.

As symptoms become more moderate in intensity, one can consider lubiprostone when constipation is predominant and alosetron when diarrhea is present. These agents are thought to have a role in achieving pain benefit independent of their effects on bowel habit. Early studies are showing some benefit for the use of antibiotics and possibly probiotics in selected patients, particularly for symptoms of bloating and abdominal discomfort (see Chapter 37).

PSYCHOTROPIC AGENTS

When pain intensity is more moderate to severe in nature, antidepressants should be considered in order to achieve both peripheral and central analgesic effects.[3] Rationale for their use in low doses relates to their effects on reducing afferent signals from the gut, modulating bowel symptoms, and enhancing descending CNS inhibition of visceral input to the brain. Higher dosages are also used when psychiatric comorbidities are present that can aggravate the pain.

The emerging concept of neuroplasticity with loss of cortical neurons in psychiatric trauma and neurogenesis (ie, regrowth of neurons) with clinical treatment provides an even greater rationale for the use of central treatments. With post-traumatic stress disorders (PTSDs), there is neuronal death in key areas, such as the dentate ganglion of the hippocampus, and recent fMRI studies now show reduced neuron density in other areas of the brain including cortical regions involved in emotional and pain regulation in patients with chronic pain including IBS. Notably, recent data suggest that antidepressant (and possibly psychological) treatments may restore lost neurons. Levels of brain-derived neurotrophic factor, a precursor of neurogenesis, increase with antidepressant treatment and correlate with longer periods of treatment and with the degree of recovery from depression. These findings provide insight into how the CNS functions in response to emotional trauma and its associations with chronic visceral and somatic pain and their treatments.

The tricyclic antidepressants (TCAs) (eg, desipramine, nortriptyline, and amitriptyline) or the new serotonin norepinepherine reuptake inhibitors (SNRIs) (duloxetine, venlafaxine, and desvenlafaxine) are of particular value in treating chronic pain syndromes owing to their combined noradrenergic and serotonergic effects. These agents have generally been more successful than selective serotonin reuptake inhibitors (SSRIs), the latter being more useful for treating associated psychiatric comorbidities such as anxiety, depression, and obsessional symptoms and in targeting global symptoms and coping rather than pain. Low doses of TCAs and SNRIs (eg, desipramine 25 to 75 mg at night or duloxetine 30 mg in the daytime) can be initiated and increased to full dosages if needed, particularly when depression is also present, and continued for 6 to 12 months or longer if needed. Narcotic analgesics should be weaned because of the possibility of developing narcotic bowel syndrome.[4]

Augmentation strategies can be useful for patients with refractory pain symptoms that are not responsive to single antidepressants or other treatments. Most gastroenterologists are not familiar with this method of treatment, but because such strategies are commonly used in psychiatry, a psychiatric consultation to plan treatment is recommended. Thus, patients who are refractory to usual dosages of antidepressants or who are experiencing side effects should be offered additional psychotropic medication to augment the clinical effect, because they act on different neuroreceptors. Recently, we have used a low-dose atypical antipsychotic agent (eg, quetiapine 25-100 mg) that acts on dopamine receptors for augmenting the antidepressant treatment in our patients with severe, refractory IBS with benefit. This class of agents has antianxiety and sleep benefits and may also have independent analgesic effects. Table 48-5 lists steps in choosing a particular psychotherapeutic agent and the approach to care of patients with FGIDs.

Gabapentin and pregabalin are increasingly being prescribed for chronic neuropathic pain conditions including peripheral neuropathies and, more recently, fibromyalgia.

Table 48-5

Choosing a Particular Psychotherapeutic Agent and the Approach to Care of Patients With IBS

1. Choice of the agent
   Specific symptom to be treated
   Side effect profile
   Cost of the drug
   Previous experiences and preferences with psychotropic agents
   Co-existing psychiatric conditions targeted

2. Initiating treatment
   Negotiate treatment plan
   Consider previous drugs that worked
   Start with a low dose (eg, 25 mg/day of TCA)

3. Continuing treatment
   Escalate dose by 25% to 50% every 1 to 2 weeks to receive therapeutic effect with minimum possible dose
   Watch for side effects—counsel that most of these disappear in 1 to 2 weeks. If they do not, try to continue same or lower dose from same class before switching to a different class
   Follow-up within first week and then within 2 to 3 weeks to ensure adherence
   Gauge treatment benefit with improvement in coping, daily function, quality of life, and emotional state
   If a poor initial response:
   Readdress patient concerns
   Switch to a different class of antidepressant
   Combine treatments as augmentation (eg, SSRI + TCA, SSRI + buspirone, pharmacological, and psychological treatment)
   If needed, obtain psychiatry consultation for pharmacotherapy
   Increase doses up to full psychiatric doses before discontinuing if patient can tolerate
   If there is no benefit in 6 to 8 weeks on higher doses, alternate strategies (eg, adding psychological treatment or referral) should be considered
   Depending upon the response and side effects, another agent with a different mechanism of action can be added to augment treatment efficacy and minimize side effects

4. Stopping treatment: Continue treatment at minimum effective doses for 6 to 12 months. Long-term therapy may be warranted for some patients. Gradually tapering to prevent withdrawal symptoms.

Their benefit for visceral or central pain syndromes are not established, although a few case reports have suggested benefit for visceral pain. These remain potential options for the treatment of pain associated with IBS and certainly should be considered if there appears to be a component of abdominal wall pain as well.

PSYCHOLOGICAL THERAPY

Interventions of potential benefit include cognitive behavioral therapy, dynamic or interpersonal psychotherapy, hypnotherapy, and stress management. Referral to pain treatment centers for multidisciplinary treatment programs may be the most efficient method of treating disability from refractory chronic pain. These treatments may not improve the pain as much as the patient's adaptation to the pain and enhancement of coping strategies ("the pain is still there but it doesn't bother me as much"). Their effects are additive to other medical treatments, the benefit continues after the treatment period ends, there are no medical side effects, and treatment may reduce healthcare costs. Critical to implementing psychological treatment is that the referring physician must help the patient accept the value of these treatments as part of their ongoing plan of care.

Summary

IBS is a common GI disorder. Abdominal pain is an important feature of IBS and the most common reason IBS patients seek out medical attention. Managing pain depends on the severity of symptoms. With mild, infrequent symptoms in the absence of psychosocial factors, managing the predominant bowel symptom can help with the pain. However, with severe symptoms, commonly associated with the presence of psychosocial disturbances, centrally acting treatments using psychotropic and behavioral strategies are usually required. In addition, the, power of an effective physician-patient relationship should be the basis of any treatment strategy.

References

1. Longstreth GF, Thompson WG, Chey WD, Houghton LA, Mearin F, Spiller RC. Functional bowel disorders. *Gastroenterology.* 2006;130:1480-1491.
2. Drossman DA, Whitehead WE, Toner BB, et al. What determines severity among patients with painful functional bowel disorders? *Am J Gastroenterol.* 2000;95:974-980.
3. Grover M, Drossman DA. Psychopharmacologic and behavioral treatments for functional gastrointestinal disorders. *Gastrointest Endosc Clin N Am.* 2009;19:151-170.
4. Grunkemeier DM, Cassara JE, Dalton CB, Drossman DA. The narcotic bowel syndrome: clinical features, pathophysiology, and management. *Clin Gastroenterol Hepatol.* 2007;5:1126-1139.

SECTION VI

WHAT DOES THE
FUTURE HOLD?

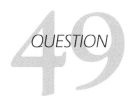
WHAT MEDICATIONS ARE ON THE HORIZON FOR THE TREATMENT OF IBS?

Michael Camilleri, MD

The pathophysiological mechanisms of irritable bowel syndrome (IBS) are not completely understood, but alterations in gastrointestinal motility, secretion, bacterial ecology, and possibly bile acid malabsorption and low grade inflammation provide a basis for the development of more effective therapies for IBS. Agents on the horizon with promise have shown a positive impact on motility, sensory, or secretory biomarkers or symptom-based efficacy in Phase IIb or Phase III trials. These agents are new-generation 5-hydroxytryptamine receptor 4 (5-HT$_4$) agonists, intestinal secretagogues (chloride channel activators, guanylate cyclase C (GC-C) agonists), and drugs approved for other indications that may be efficacious in IBS including bile acid modulators, anti-inflammatory agents, and visceral analgesics.

New-generation 5-HT$_4$ agonists are selective with high intrinsic activity for intestinal 5-HT$_4$ receptors, devoid of effects on the hERG (human ether-a-go-go related gene) channel, and without clinically meaningful effects on 5-HT$_4$ receptors in the heart. These medications include prucalopride, ATI-7505 (naronapride), and velusetrag. Prucalopride was approved by the European Medicines Agency (EMEA) in October 2009 for the symptomatic treatment of chronic constipation in women based on consistent efficacy in three pivotal Phase III trials (≥ 3 spontaneous and complete bowel movements [SCBMs] per week, increase of ≥ 1 SCBM per week, and satisfaction on a patient's assessment of constipation quality of life: PAC-QOL). Prucalopride is well-tolerated. The most common adverse events are headache, nausea, abdominal pain, and diarrhea, occurring in approximately 10% of treated participants and mainly on day 1 of treatment. With a cumulative experience of more than 1000 patient-years in open trials, no significant safety signal was identified. The approved daily dose in Europe is 2 mg in adults and 1 mg in those over 65 years of age.

Velusetrag (TD-5108) demonstrated clinical efficacy in a pharmacodynamic transit study with accelerated overall colonic transit and ascending colon emptying and in a Phase IIB trial of 401 patients with chronic constipation. The most promising doses are 15 and 30 mg/day.

Ramosetron is a potent and selective synthetic **5-HT3 receptor antagonist** with efficacy in patients with diarrhea-predominant IBS (IBS-D), at once-daily doses of 5 and 10 µg. The incidence of constipation is lower than with alosetron. Further studies are necessary to elucidate if the risk of ischemic colitis differentiates this drug from alosetron.

Two classes of **secretagogues** have opened a new avenue for management of lower FGID. Chloride ion (Cl⁻) transport regulates fluid secretion into the intestine; Cl⁻ movement across the apical membrane is via the cyclic adenosine monophosphate (cAMP)-dependent cystic fibrosis transmembrane regulator (CFTR) chloride channel and the type 2 Cl⁻ channel (ClC-2). *Lubiprostone* is approved by FDA for the treatment of chronic constipation and IBS-C. Lubiprostone enhances intestinal fluid secretion, resulting in accelerated small intestinal and colonic transit, and relieves C-IBS (16 µg/day) and chronic constipation (48 µg/day). The most common adverse event is nausea (see Chapter 38).

Linaclotide is a guanylate cyclase C (GC-C) agonist that induces intestinal Cl⁻ secretion through the CFTR channel. In women with C-IBS, linaclotide significantly accelerated ascending colonic transit and altered bowel function, increasing the number of bowel movements and loosening stool consistency. Beneficial clinical effects were demonstrated in Phase IIB and III randomized controlled trials in chronic constipation and in Phase IIB trials in IBS-C (see Chapter 43).

Among **centrally acting agents**, the benzodiazepine receptor modulator *dextofisopam* was superior to placebo in a double-blind, placebo-controlled study of patients with diarrhea-predominant or alternating IBS, particularly during the first 4 weeks of treatment, with adequate relief and improved consistency and frequency of bowel movements. Further studies are required.

Medications Approved for Other Indications Are Being Tested in IBS

Disruption of the enterohepatic circulation of **bile acids** due to ileal disease induces fluid secretion in the human colon. Randomized, double-blind, placebo-controlled studies demonstrated that ileocolonic delivery of chenodeoxycholate (CDC) at doses of 500 and 1000 mg/day accelerated colonic transit and loosened stool consistency in healthy volunteers and in patients with IBS-C. On the other hand, up to 70% of patients with chronic watery diarrhea have bile acid (BA) malabsorption; BA binding relieves chronic diarrhea. The well-tolerated bile acid binding agent, colesevelam hydrochloride, delayed overall colonic transit and emptying of the ascending colon, inducing greater ease of stool passage and somewhat firmer stool consistency.

A subgroup of patients with IBS has subtle inflammatory changes in colonic biopsies, thus providing the rationale for testing **anti-inflammatory agents** and mast-cell stabilizers in IBS. *Disodium cromoglycate* (DSCG) resulted in clinical improvement of bowel function in a pilot study of seven IBS-D patients. *Ketotifen*, a mast cell stabilizer, increased the threshold for discomfort in 30 visceral hypersensitive IBS patients and decreased the percentage of patients reporting severe abdominal pain, bloating, flatulence, diarrhea, and improved quality of life subscales of sleep, diet, and sexual functioning. Sedation or drowsiness was observed in the patients receiving ketotifen. *5-aminosalicylic acid* was tested in a pilot trial of 20 patients with IBS; it significantly reduced inflammation and was associated with improved general well-being, but primary colonic symptoms did not significantly change.

Among **visceral analgesics**, *asimadoline*, a peripheral kappa opioid-agonist, inhibited perception of visceral sensation with no effect on GI transit or colonic contractile responses. In a randomized, double-blind, placebo-controlled trial, asimadoline produced improvement in symptoms in IBS-D patients who had at least moderate pain at baseline. Intermittent use of asimadoline during attacks of IBS pain was not found to be efficacious. *Pregabalin* is approved for treatment of fibromyalgia and neuropathic pain. It was shown to reduce visceral sensation, and it is currently undergoing clinical trials.

Summary

There has been exciting progress in the development of novel agents to treat IBS, including treatments originally used for different indications, such as bile acid binding, and anti-inflammatory agents. We still need to identify clinical strategies to individualize treatment based on the underlying pathophysiology. Until that happens, treatment of IBS will remain a hit-or-miss affair despite the pharmacological qualities, proven pharmacodynamic efficacy, and safety evaluations of promising new therapies for IBS.

Bibliography

Camilleri M. Review article: new receptor targets for medical therapy in irritable bowel syndrome. *Aliment Pharmacol Ther.* 2010;31:35-46.

Camilleri M, Chang L. Challenges to the therapeutic pipeline for irritable bowel syndrome: end points and regulatory hurdles. *Gastroenterology.* 2008;135:1877-1891.

Camilleri M, Kerstens R, Rykx A, et al. A placebo-controlled trial of prucalopride for severe chronic constipation. *N Engl J Med.* 2008;358:2344-2354.

Spiller R, Camilleri M, Longstreth GF. Do the symptom-based, Rome criteria of irritable bowel syndrome lead to better diagnosis and treatment outcomes? *Clin Gastroenterol Hepatol.* 2010;8:125-129; discussion 129-136.

Acknowledgment: I thank Mrs. Cindy Stanislav for her excellent secretarial support.

FINANCIAL DISCLOSURES

Dr. Giovanni Barbara has not disclosed any relevant financial relationships.

Dr. Adil E. Bharucha has not disclosed any relevant financial relationships.

Dr. Steven J. Bollipo has not disclosed any relevant financial relationships.

Dr. Michael Camilleri has received research grants related to the subject matter of this chapter from Microbia, Theravance, and ARYx. He also serves as a consultant to Ironwood, ARYx, and Theravance, earning less than the federal threshold for significant financial conflict of interest as an aggregate from the three companies together. Dr. Camilleri has signed a confidentiality disclosure agreement with Movetis to have access to prucalopride data, but does not receive any financial remuneration.

Dr. Brooks D. Cash has not disclosed any relevant financial relationships.

Dr. Joseph Y. Chang has not disclosed any relevant financial relationships.

Dr. Lin Chang has not disclosed any relevant financial relationships.

Dr. Rok Seon Choung has not disclosed any relevant financial relationships.

Dr. Filippo Cremonini has not disclosed any relevant financial relationships.

Dr. Michael D. Crowell has not disclosed any relevant financial relationships.

Dr. Douglas A. Drossman has not disclosed any relevant financial relationships.

Dr. Ronnie Fass is a consultant, researcher, and speaker for Takeda Pharmaceuticals. She is a consultant for GlaxoSmithKline, for Vector, for Xenoport, and a consultant and speaker for Eisai.

Dr. Fernando Fernández-Bañares has no financial relationships to disclose.

Dr. Alexander Ford has not disclosed any relevant financial relationships.

Dr. Amy E. Foxx Orenstein has not disclosed any relevant financial relationships.

Dr. Elizabeth A. Friedlander has not disclosed any relevant financial relationships.

Dr. Christine Frissora has not disclosed any relevant financial relationships.

Dr. Larissa Fujii has not disclosed any relevant financial relationships.

Dr. Madhusudan Grover has not disclosed any relevant financial relationships.

Dr. Kok-Ann Gwee has not disclosed any relevant financial relationships.

Dr. Albena Halpert has not disclosed any relevant financial relationships.

Dr. Lucinda A. Harris has not disclosed any relevant financial relationships.

Dr. Margaret M. Heitkemper has not disclosed any relevant financial relationships.

Dr. Tiberiu Hershcovici has not disclosed any relevant financial relationships.

Dr. Lesley A. Houghton has not disclosed any relevant financial relationships.

Dr. Basma Issa has not disclosed any relevant financial relationships.

Dr. John E. Kellow has no financial relationships to disclose.

Dr. David Klibansky has not disclosed any relevant financial relationships.

Dr. Jeff Lackner has not disclosed any relevant financial relationships.

Dr. Anthony Lembo has not disclosed any relevant financial relationships.

Dr. L. Campbell Levy has not disclosed any relevant financial relationships.

Dr. Rona L. Levy has not disclosed any relevant financial relationships.

Dr. G. Richard Locke has not disclosed any relevant financial relationships.

Dr. Burr Loew has not disclosed any relevant financial relationships.

Dr. Susan Lucak has not disclosed any relevant financial relationships.

Dr. Tisha N. Lunsford has not disclosed any relevant financial relationships.

Dr. Juan Malagelada has not disclosed any relevant financial relationships.

Dr. Kalyani Meduri has not disclosed any relevant financial relationships.

Dr. Anil Minocha has not disclosed any relevant financial relationships.

Dr. Paul Moayyedi has not disclosed any relevant financial relationships.

Dr. Rupa Mukherjee has not disclosed any relevant financial relationships.

Dr. Agata Mulak has not disclosed any relevant financial relationships.

Dr. Richard Nahas has not disclosed any relevant financial relationships.

Dr. Kevin W. Olden has not disclosed any relevant financial relationships.

Dr. Peter Paine has not disclosed any relevant financial relationships.

Dr. Mark Pimentel has not disclosed any relevant financial relationships.

Dr. Eamonn M. M. Quigley has not disclosed any relevant financial relationships.

Dr. Chris Radziwon has no financial relationships to disclose.

Dr. Satish S. C. Rao has not disclosed any relevant financial relationships.

Dr. Yehuda Ringel has not disclosed any relevant financial relationships.

Dr. Gisela Ringström has no financial relationships to disclose.

Dr. Yuri A. Saito-Loftus has not disclosed any relevant financial relationships.

Dr. Lawrence R. Schiller has not disclosed any relevant financial relationships.

Dr. Max J. Schmulson has not disclosed any relevant financial relationships.

Dr. Philip Schoenfeld has not disclosed any relevant financial relationships.

Dr. Ankur Sheth has not disclosed any relevant financial relationships.

Dr. Lisa Shim has not disclosed any relevant financial relationships.

Dr. Corey A. Siegel has not disclosed any relevant financial relationships.

Dr. Magnus Simrén has not disclosed any relevant financial relationships.

Dr. Ami D. Sperber has no financial relationships to disclose.

Dr. Brennan Spiegel has not disclosed any relevant financial relationships.

Dr. Vincenzo Stanghellini has not disclosed any relevant financial relationships.

Dr. Yvette Taché has not disclosed any relevant financial relationships.

Dr. Jan Tack has not disclosed any relevant financial relationships.

Dr. Nicholas J. Talley has not disclosed any relevant financial relationships.

Dr. W. Grant Thompson has not disclosed any relevant financial relationships.

Dr. Kirsten T. Weiser has not disclosed any relevant financial relationships.

Dr. Peter J. Whorwell has not disclosed any relevant financial relationships.

INDEX

Printed in the United States
by Baker & Taylor Publisher Services